O A U L
OXFORD AMERICAN UROLOGY LIBRARY

Erectile Dysfunction

This material is not intended to be, and should not be considered, a substitute for medical or other professional advice. Treatment for the conditions described in this material is highly dependent on the individual circumstances. While this material is designed to offer accurate information with respect to the subject matter covered and to be current as of the time it was written, research and knowledge about medical and health issues are constantly evolving, and dose schedules for medications are being revised continually, with new side effects recognized and accounted for regularly. Readers must therefore always check the product information and clinical procedures with the most up-to-date published product information and data sheets provided by the manufacturers and the most recent codes of conduct and safety regulation. Oxford University Press and the authors make no representations or warranties to readers, express or implied, as to the accuracy or completeness of this material, including without limitation that they make no representations or warranties as to the accuracy or efficacy of the drug dosages mentioned in the material. The authors and the publishers do not accept, and expressly disclaim, any responsibility for any liability, loss, or risk that may be claimed or incurred as a consequence of the use and/or application of any of the contents of this material.

The Publisher is responsible for author selection and the Publisher and the Author(s) make all editorial decisions, including decisions regarding content. The Publisher and the Author(s) are not responsible for any product information added to this publication by companies purchasing copies of it for distribution to clinicians.

O A U L

OXFORD AMERICAN UROLOGY LIBRARY

Erectile Dysfunction

Edited by

Ernst R. Schwarz, MD, PhD

California Medical Institute
Beverly Hills, Temecula, and Los Angeles, California
and
Cedars-Sinai Medical Center/
University of California – Los Angeles
Los Angeles, California

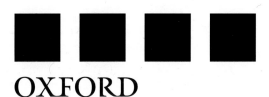

OXFORD
UNIVERSITY PRESS

OXFORD
UNIVERSITY PRESS

Oxford University Press is a department of the University of Oxford.
It furthers the University's objective of excellence in research, scholarship,
and education by publishing worldwide.

Oxford   New York
Auckland   Cape Town   Dar es Salaam   Hong Kong   Karachi
Kuala Lumpur   Madrid   Melbourne   Mexico City   Nairobi
New Delhi   Shanghai   Taipei   Toronto

With offices in
Argentina   Austria   Brazil   Chile   Czech Republic   France   Greece
Guatemala   Hungary   Italy   Japan   Poland   Portugal   Singapore
South Korea   Switzerland   Thailand   Turkey   Ukraine   Vietnam

Oxford is a registered trademark of Oxford University Press in the UK
and certain other countries.

Published in the United States of America by
Oxford University Press
198 Madison Avenue, New York, NY 10016

Library of Congress Cataloging-in-Publication Data
Erectile dysfunction / [edited by] Ernst R. Schwarz.
    p. ; cm.—(Oxford American urology library)
Includes bibliographical references and index.
ISBN 978–0-19–979489–8 (alk. paper)
I. Schwarz, Ernst R. II. Series: Oxford American urology library.
[DNLM: 1. Erectile Dysfunction.   2. Risk Factors. WJ 709]
616.6922—dc23
2012042896

ISBN-13: 978–0–19–979489–8

9 8 7 6 5 4 3 2 1
Printed in the United States of America
on acid-free paper

Preface

Erectile dysfunction (ED) is usually considered a vascular disease that affects approximately at least 30 million American adult men, mainly above the age of 50 years. The causes are often multifactorial and include exposure to common vascular risk factors such as diabetes, hypertension, hyperlipidemia, and smoking, among others, leading to endothelial dysfunction. Similarly, other than penile vascular territories can be affected, indicating a generalized vascular pathology that might present first with ED. As such, a multidisciplinary approach is warranted to ensure adequate risk factor reduction, diagnostic evaluation, as well as treatment of erectile and generalized endothelial dysfunction, which not only impairs men's quality of life but also represents a potential cause for future cardiovascular events such as cerebral strokes and myocardial and peripheral ischemia. Therefore, not only urologists but also internists and cardiologists, among other specialists, are confronted with and interested in the evaluation and management of ED. Since satisfactory sexual activity is a major part of individual health, well-being, and quality of life, individuals' and the public's expectation for appropriate medical management to improve impaired sexual performance is of growing importance. In particular, patients with chronic and often incurable diseases such as diabetes, renal failure, atherosclerosis, and heart failure request and deserve medical attention to address ED that often is worsened by medications and not adequately addressed by physicians and health care providers in view of other pertinent medical problems.

As an example, a few years ago I discussed with colleagues the issue of sexual dysfunction in patients who received a left ventricular assist device for end-stage heart failure, either as a bridge to cardiac transplantation or as so-called 'destination therapy'. The overall response I received was that these patients are so sick that they would not even think about sexual activity. Fact is, as it turned out in an internal survey, most of our patients were between the ages of 30 and 70 years, and questions about sexual functioning and activity were actually expressed by at least 80% of our patients.

It was the aim of this book on ED to look beyond the prescription of PDE-5 inhibitors and to evaluate and manage men with ED using a multidisciplinary approach. Therefore, I invited opinion leaders around the country from urology, cardiology, vascular medicine, psychiatry, internal medicine, transplant medicine, basic and clinical research, and age management to contribute to the chapters of this book. It should encourage all of us health care providers and scientists to emphasize the importance of ED for health and well-being.

Ernst R. Schwarz, MD, PhD
Beverly Hills, April 2013

Contents

Contributors

Brian H. Annex, MD
Division of Cardiovascular Medicine
University of Virginia Health System
Charlottesville, Virginia

Konstantin Balayan, MD
David Geffen School of Medicine
Cedars-Sinai Medical Center/
University of California – Los Angeles
Los Angeles, California

Anthony J. Bella MD FRCSC
Greta and John Hansen Chair in
    Men's Health Research
Assistant Professor of Urology,
    Department of Surgery
Associate Scientist, Neuroscience
University of Ottawa
Ontario, Canada

Raymond M. Bernal, MD
Division of Urology, Department of
    Surgery
Duke University
Durham, North Carolina

Ellen R. Goldmark, MD
Resident, Division of Urology
University of Maryland Medical
    Center
Baltimore, Maryland

Jason C. Huang, MD
Resident, Department of Internal
    Medicine
University of Virginia Health System
Charlottesville, Virginia

**Waguih William IsHak, MD,
FAPA**
Associate Clinical Professor,
    Psychiatry and Biobehavioral
    Sciences
David Geffen School of Medicine
Cedars-Sinai Medical Center/
University of California – Los Angeles
Los Angeles, California

Ashraf Ismail, MD
David Geffen School of Medicine
Cedars-Sinai Medical Center/
University of California –
    Los Angeles
Los Angeles, California

Mohit Khera, MD, MBA, MPH
Assistant Professor of Urology
Baylor College of Medicine
Houston, Texas

Robert A. Kloner MD, PhD
The Heart Institute, Good Samaritan
    Hospital
Division of Cardiology, Keck School
    of Medicine
University of Southern
    California
Los Angeles, California

Andrew C. Kramer, MD
Associate Professor of Surgery,
    Division of Urology
University
Maryland Medical Center
Baltimore, Maryland

CONTRIBUTORS

Martin M. Miner MD
Co-Director Men's Health Center
The Miriam Hospital
Clinical Associate Professor of Family
    Medicine
The Warren Alpert School of Medicine
Brown University
Providence, Rhode Island

Anita Phan, MD
California Medical Institute and
    Cedars Sinai Medical Center,
Beverly Hills and Los Angeles,
    California

Thorsten Reffelmann MD
Klinik und Poliklinik für Innere
    Medizin B
Universitätsklinikum der Ernst-Moritz-
    Arndt-Universität Greifswald
Greifswald, Germany

Ernst R. Schwarz, MD, PhD
California Medical Institute
Beverly Hills and Los Angeles,
    California, and

Cedars-Sinai Medical Center/
    University of California –
    Los Angeles
Los Angeles, California

Rany Shamloul
Division of Urology, Department of
    Surgery,
University of Ottawa
    Ontario, Canada, and
Department of Andrology
Cairo University
Cairo, Egypt

Paul D. Thompson, MD
President, Cenegenics DFW
Arlington, Texas

Dioma U. Udeoji, MD
California Medical Institute,
    Beverly Hills and Los Angeles,
    and Cedars Sinai
    Medical Center,
Los Angeles, California

Chapter 1

Erectile Dysfunction: The Scope of the Problem of Sexual Dysfunction in Men

Ernst R. Schwarz

Definition

As defined by the National Institute of Health (NIH), erectile dysfunction (ED) is the repeated inability to get an erection firm enough for sexual intercourse (1). The International Consultation on Sexual Medicine defined ED as the consistent or recurrent inability to attain and/or maintain penile erection sufficient for sexual performance (2). These definitions exclude other causes of sexual dysfunction, including decreased libido and premature ejaculation.

Historical Perspective

Impotence has been studied for hundreds of years, but not until the past few decades have we been able to understand and treat it so effectively. Even in the early 1900s there was the knowledge that the vascular, neurological, and hormonal milieu played a part in erections, as physicians performed dorsal vein ligations and testicular transplants. However, the complex physiological, neurological, and psychological interaction is only just starting to be appreciated. Up until the 1980s, most ED cases were still attributed to psychological factors. This was due largely in part to the influence of Freud and his views that impotence was caused by the well-known Oedipal complex. In the era before pharmacological treatment, most men with ED were assumed to have psychosexual issues that were then diagnosed and treated by psychologists and psychiatrists. With the dawn of pharmacological treatment in the 1980s and advances in ultrasound techniques, physicians were able to create erections and monitor blood flow into and out of the penis and have a way of measuring the efficacy of treatment. Intracavernosal therapy was the primary and most efficacious treatment at that time until the discovery of nitric oxide and its role in erection physiology.

Pharmacological treatment changes as we understand more about the etiology of ED. It has been 12 years since the U.S. Food & Drug Administration (FDA) approved sildenafil (Viagra), an oral phosphodiesterase inhibitor, and there is a new algorithm of treatment that centers on the patient's goals and motivations and evidence-based principles (3). Over 70% of ED cases can now be treated with oral medications. Oral pharmacotherapy is the first-line treatment for almost all types of ED according to the American Urological Association/European Urological Association guidelines and the World Health Organization-sponsored International Consultation on treatment for erectile dysfunction (4–6). This brought the diagnosis and treatment of ED to the fore-front of medicine and made it a household discussion.

Prevalence and Incidence

According to most recent studies, somewhere between 15 and 30 million men report sexual dysfunction in the United States. There has also been an increase in self-reported ED according to the National Ambulatory Medical Care Survey, as men are seeking simple treatments such as oral phosphodiesterase inhibitors (7). A systematic review done in 2002 found that the prevalence of ED world-wide ranges from 2% in those less than 40 years of age to over 80% in men over 80 (8). This review looked at studies in Europe, Asia, the United States, and Australia. One of the difficulties with determining the prevalence of ED is the differences in reporting ED, cultural perceptions of ED, and understanding of comorbidities worldwide.

What we do know is that ED is associated with aging and with other med-ical conditions. The Massachusetts Male Aging Study (MMAS) was one of the first large population-based studies showing that the prevalence of ED was associated with aging, while also showing the association with other chronic illnesses such as diabetes mellitus, hyperlipidemia, obesity, hypertension, and depression (9). The results from this study showed that the prevalence of ED increased from 39% for men in their 40s to 67% for men over 70. More recently, the Cross-National Survey on Male Health Issues was a study that used the same questionnaire as the MMAS but included the United States, Germany, the United Kingdom, Italy, France, and Spain. The overall prevalence of ED was 19% and the largest variable to correlate with ED was age (10). Across the six countries, the prevalence ranged from 4% to 6% in men younger than 40 to 39% to 73% in men older than 70. Other studies that have independently been done in Germany, France, Spain, Japan, and Malaysia show similar rates of prevalence and an age-dependent increase of ED, while taking into account the limitations of cross-cultural studies (11–14).

Risk Factors

The cause of ED may be vasculogenic, neurogenic, endocrine, psychogenic, or of mixed etiology. This gives a wide range of risk factors, including modifiable lifestyle choices, genetic predisposition, and even iatrogenic causes.

As previously highlighted, the largest risk factor for ED is aging, as dem-onstrated by multiple epidemiological studies. Other identifiable risk fac-tors include smoking, heart disease, diabetes, renal failure, hyperlipidemia, depression, obesity, and trauma. Neurological diseases that can cause ED include spinal cord injury, multiple sclerosis, and Parkinson's disease. Recent evidence has shown that not only is heart disease a risk factor for ED, but ED may be a precursor to heart disease and the diagnosis of ED may precede the onset of cardiac events (15, 16). The MMAS study also demonstrated that the incidence of ED is three times greater in diabetic versus nondiabetic patients and is diagnosed at an earlier age in people with diabetes than in the general public (9, 17).

When a risk factor is identified in the history, it is important to point that out to the patient as a potential source for the ED and offer suggestions to modify lifestyle. The incidence of cigarette smoking was not higher in cases of ED in the MMAS group; however, many other studies show an increased risk of ED in men who smoke, and smoking is clearly associated with heart disease, which is associated with ED (18, 19).

Obesity, exercise, and diet also have been implicated in ED. Studies have shown that making improvements in certain areas of lifestyle can improve erectile function. Esposito and colleagues in 2004 demonstrated that weight loss improves men's perceptions of their ED (20). In addition to chronic illnesses that are risk factors for ED, many of the medications used to treat heart disease, hypertension, and neurological disorders can cause ED. It has been reported that up to 60% of men taking antidepressants and 20% taking antihypertensives have experienced ED (21).

Other major risk factors for ED are surgery and trauma. Especially now, as the primary treatment for prostate cancer is still radical prostatectomy, up to 50% of men may experience ED after surgery. A thorough surgical history should include any previous perineal, pelvic, or genital trauma. Up to 30% of pelvic fractures may result in ED secondary to vascular or neurological injury (22). Other surgeries in addition to prostatectomy that can cause ED include cystoprostatectomy, abdominoperineal resection, renal transplantation, and vascular surgery.

ED is clearly multifactorial, but by recognizing the risk factors we can have better conversations with our patients about appropriate treatments and interventions.

Impact of ED

The effects of ED go beyond just sexual function and have implications for quality of life (QoL), development of comorbid conditions, and interpersonal relationships.

Few studies have measured QoL associated with ED. While we know that depression is associated with ED and may be caused by ED, other factors related to QoL have been more difficult to ascertain. A few studies have assessed satisfaction with the use of intraurethral Medicated Urethral System for Erection (MUSE™) injection of alprostadil, and these showed improvement with partner relationships and personal wellness (23, 24). Other studies have looked at ED in men after prostate cancer therapy and have documented decreased QoL outcomes in men both with and without prostate cancer (25). The International

Index of Erectile Dysfunction (IIEF) contains questions pertaining to overall satisfaction and the man's relationship with his partner (26).

While the use of oral medications has increased substantially and can treat up to 70% of ED cases, studies have shown that there is only about a 20% to 50% refill rate for prescriptions for the phosphodiesterase inhibitors (27, 28). This alludes to the fact that while ED does affect QoL, there are multiple factors that contribute to choice of treatment and adherence to treatment (29). While ED is extremely common, there is still a lot of research to be done in terms of preventive measures, finding better treatments, and identifying treatment outcomes on QoL.

References

1. NIH Consensus Conference. Impotence. NIH Consensus Development Panel on Impotence. *JAMA* 1993;270:83–90.

2. Jardin A. *Recommendations of the 1st International Consultation on Erectile Dysfunction.* Plymouth, UK: Health Publications Ltd., 2000.

3. Rosen RC, Hatzichristou D, Broderick G. Clinical evaluation and symptom scales: Sexual dysfunction assessment in men. In Lue T, Basson R, Rosen R, eds. *Sexual Medicine: Sexual Dysfunctions in Men and Women.* Paris: Health Publications, 2004.

4. Lue TF. Erectile dysfunction. *N Engl J Med* 2000;342(24):1802–1813.

5. Montague DK. The management of erectile dysfunction: an AUA update. *J Urol* 2005;174(1):230–239.

6. Wespes E et al. EAU Guidelines on erectile dysfunction: an update. *Eur Urol* 2006;49(5):806–815.

7. Wessells H et al. Erectile dysfunction. *J Urol* 2007;177:1675–1681.

8. Prins J et al. Prevalence of erectile dysfunction: a systematic review of population-based studies. *Int J Impot Res* 2002;14(6):422–432.

9. Feldman HA et al. Impotence and its medical and psychosocial correlates: results of the Massachusetts Male Aging Study. *J Urol* 1994;151:54–61.

10. Shabsigh R et al. Drivers and barriers to seeking treatment for erectile dysfunction: a comparison of six countries. *BJU Int* 2004;94(7):1055–1065.

11. Martin-Morales A et al. Prevalence and independent risk factors for erectile dysfunction in Spain: results of the Epidemiologia de la Disfuncion Erectil Masculina Study. *J Urol* 2001;166(2):569–575.

12. Giuliano F et al. Prevalence of erectile dysfunction in France: results of an epidemiological survey of a representative sample of 1004 men. *Eur Urol* 2002;42(4):382–389.

13. Braun M et al. Epidemiology of erectile dysfunction: results of the Cologne Male Survey. *Int J Impot Res* 2000;12(6):305–311.

14. Nicolosi A et al. Epidemiology of erectile dysfunction in four countries: cross-national study of the prevalence and correlates of erectile dysfunction. *Urology* 2003;61(1):201–206.

15. Burchardt M et al. Erectile dysfunction is a marker for cardiovascular complications and psychological functioning in men with hypertension. *Int J Impot Res* 2001;13(5):276–281.

16. Kirby MG et al. Prevalence and detection rate of underlying disease in men with erectile dysfunction receiving phosphodiesterase type 5 inhibitors in the United Kingdom: a retrospective database study. *Int J Clin Pract* 2011;65(7):797–806.

17. Shabsigh R et al. Health issues of men: prevalence and correlates of erectile dysfunction. *J Urol* 2005;174(2): 662–667.

18. Mirone V et al. Cigarette smoking as risk factor for erectile dysfunction: results from an Italian epidemiological study. *Eur Urol* 2002;41(3):294–297.

19. Shabsigh R et al. Cigarette smoking and other vascular risk factors in vasculogenic impotence. *Urology* 1991;38(3):227–231.

20. Esposito K et al. Effect of lifestyle changes on erectile dysfunction in obese men: a randomized controlled trial. *JAMA* 2004;291:2978–2984.

21. Meuleman EJ. Prevalence of erectile dysfunction: need for treatment? *Int J Impot Res* 2002;14(Suppl 1):S22–28.

22. Shenfeld OZ et al. The incidence and causes of erectile dysfunction after pelvic fractures associated with posterior urethral disruption. *J Urol* 2003;169(6):2173–2176.

23. Williams G et al. The effect of transurethral alprostadil on the quality of life of men with erectile dysfunction, and their partners. MUSE Study Group. *Br J Urol* 1998;82(6):847–854.

24. Purvis K, Egdetveit I, Christiansen E. Intracavernosal therapy for erectile failure—impact of treatment and reasons for drop-out and dissatisfaction. *Int J Impot Res* 1999;11(5):287–299.

25. Penson DF et al. Is quality of life different for men with erectile dysfunction and prostate cancer compared to men with erectile dysfunction due to other causes? Results from the ExCEED data base. *J Urol* 2003;169(4):1458–1461.

26. Rosen RC et al. The International Index of Erectile Function (IIEF): a multidimensional scale for assessment of erectile dysfunction. *Urology* 1997;49:822–830.

27. Mulhall JP et al. Medication utilization behavior in patients receiving phosphodiesterase type 5 inhibitors for erectile dysfunction. *J Sex Med* 2005;2(6):848–855.

28. Sadovsky R et al. Three-year update of sildenafil citrate (Viagra) efficacy and safety. *Int J Clin Pract* 2001;55(2):115–128.

29. Perelman M et al. Attitudes of men with erectile dysfunction: a cross-national survey. *J Sex Med* 2005;2(3):397–406.

Chapter 2

Physiology of Erections and Pathophysiology of Erectile Dysfunction

Mohit Khera

Introduction

The integrated relationship between penile tumescence and detumescence is influenced by numerous central and peripheral factors, such as neurotransmitters, hormones, mechanical and other sensory stimulation, and certain disease processes. Over the past three decades our understanding of the physiology of erections and pathophysiology of ED has been significantly enhanced. Our understanding of the physiology of erections has led to the advent of numerous medications and treatments such as phosphodiesterase inhibitors, intraurethral suppositories, and intracavernosal injections. Further understanding of how certain disease processes affect erectile function has also led to strategies to prevent the development of ED.

Anatomy

The two main functions of the penis are urinary and sexual. The superficial layers of the penis include the epidermis, superficial fascia (Colles' fascia), and Buck's fascia (Fig. 2.1). The deeper structures of the penis comprise three cylinders, with the two corpora cavernosal bodies and a corpus spongiosum. The corpus spongiosum dilates distally to form the glans penis and allows the urethra to exit and allow for micturition. The corpus spongiosum originates from the perineum and is surrounded by the bulbocavernosus muscle. The corpora cavernosa are surrounded by the tunica albuginea and allow for penile rigidity during an erection. The corpora cavernosa communicate distally because of an incomplete intercavernosal septum.

The arteries to the penis originate from the internal pudendal artery, which branches from the hypogastric artery. The internal pudendal artery subdivides into the cavernosal artery, the dorsal penile artery, and the bulbo-urethral artery (which further subdivides into the urethral and bulbar arteries). The cavernous arteries branch into the helacine arteries, which open into the lacunar spaces. These sinusoidal spaces are composed of smooth

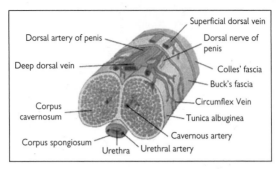

Figure 2.1 Normal penile anatomy demonstrating superficial and deep layers of the penis.

muscle and endothelium and are what ultimately provide penile rigidity. The lacunar spaces drain into venules, which drain into the subalbugineal plexus and eventually the emissary veins (1). The venous drainage of the penis is continued with the circumflex veins and the deep dorsal vein of the penis. The superficial dorsal vein drains the superficial penile tissue and is located superior to Buck's fascia.

The penis is innervated from the sympathetic fibers originating from the thoracolumbar vertebrae (T11–L2) and from sympathetic fibers from the sacrum (S2–4). The parasympathetic fibers are primarily responsible for penile tumescence, while the sympathetic fibers are responsible for penile detumescence. The penis also has somatic nerve innervations with sensory nerves and motor nerves, which are responsible for contracting the bulbocavernosous and ischiocavernosus muscles.

Physiology of Penile Erections

Mechanism of Penile Tumescence and Detumescence

Three types of erections have been defined: nocturnal, reflexogenic, and psychogenic or central. Nocturnal erections usually follow rapid eye movement sleep. Reflexogenic erections originate from genital stimulation. Central or psychogenic erections occur from stimulation of the senses, such as olfactory or visual stimuli, or erotic thoughts.

Tumescence mainly involves sinusoidal relaxation, arterial dilation, and venous compression (2). Initially, sexual stimulation results in release of neurotransmitters from the cavernous nerve terminals. This results in vasodilation of the cavernosal arteries and increased blood flow. Increased blood flow in the lacunar spaces expands the cavernous sinusoids and causes compression of the subtunical venous plexus between the tunica albuginea and the peripheral sinusoids and results in decreased venous outflow. The relaxation of the cavernous smooth muscle depends on endocrine, paracrine, and autocrine mechanisms. The stretching of the tunica albuginea occludes the emissary veins between the inner circular and outer longitudinal layers and further inhibits venous outflow. Greater intracavernosal pressures result in full erection and, finally, a rigid erection.

Detumescence occurs in three phases (3). The first phase results in a transient increase in intracorporal pressures, which signifies the beginning of smooth muscle contractions. In the second phase there is a slow pressure decrease secondary to a slow reopening of the venous channels. The last phase demonstrates a fast pressure decrease with completely restored venous outflow.

Central Mechanisms of Erections

The three areas in the central nervous system most commonly studied to obtain information about erections are the paraventricular nuclei, the medial preoptic area, and the hippocampus. These centers have been regarded as important integration centers for penile erections and libido (4). The most commonly studied central neurotransmitters involved in penile tumescence are dopamine and serotonin. Dopamine, a catecholamine that is synthesized from phenylalanine, facilitates erections in the paraventricular nucleus through D2 receptors (5). Serotonin mainly inhibits erections through the HT1A receptors. Neurons containing serotonin can be found in the ventral medulla reticular formation, the medullary raphe nuclei, and bulbospinous neurons (6). Other major inhibitors of erections include norepinephrine, gamma amino-butyric acid (GABA), prolactin, and enkephalins (5) (Table 2.1). Oxytocin also plays an important role in the autonomic nervous system. Studies have demonstrated that oxytocin is a potent inducer of penile erections when injected into the paraventricular nucleus, the lateral cerebral ventricle, and the hippocampus. These erections can be blocked by injecting oxytocin antagonists in the paraventricular nucleus or into the lateral ventricles (7–9).

Peripheral Mechanisms of Erections

Peripheral neurotransmitters are categorized as those originating from peripheral nerves and those originating from the endothelium (Table 2.2). Neurogenic neurotransmitters include nitric oxide (neuronal), vasoactive intestinal peptide (VIP), acetylcholine, and norepinephrine. Nitric oxide (NO) is the main mediator of the nonadrenergic, noncholinergic mechanism of penile erections and is synthesized from l-arginine from nitric oxide synthase (NOS) (6, 10). With sexual stimulation, NO is released into the nerve terminals and into the endothelial cells. NO facilitates conversion of GTP into cyclic GMP by means of guanylate cyclase. Cyclic GMP is in turn responsible for cavernous smooth muscle vasodilation. Contraction of human penile arteries and trabecular smooth muscle is mainly mediated by alpha-1 adrenergic receptors (11, 12). The noradrenergic pathway is responsible for detumescence after ejaculation and the basal tone of the cavernous smooth muscles during sexual inactivity. Adrenergic stimulation

Table 2.1 Central Neurotransmitters	
Excitatory	**Inhibitory**
Dopamine	Serotonin
Oxytocin	Norepinephrine
	GABA
	Prolactin
	Enkephalins

Table 2.2 Peripheral Neurotransmitters

Neuronal	Endothelium
Nitric oxide	Nitric oxide
VIP	Endothelin 1
Acetylcholine	Prostaglandin E1
Norepinephrine	

causes vasoconstriction of the penile arteries and contraction of the cavernous smooth muscle, which results in decreased arterial blood flow and subsequent increase in venous drainage (13–15).

Over the past several years the endothelium has been a major focus of strategies to improve erectile function and prevent ED. The neurotransmitters associated with the endothelium include endothelin 1, NO (endothelial), and prostaglandin E1. Endothelin-1 is synthesized by the endothelium of the lacunar spaces and is also responsible for smooth muscle vasoconstriction. Prostaglandins have been shown to have both excitatory and inhibitory effects on cavernous smooth muscle contractions. Prostaglandins are produced from arachidonic acid through the action of cyclooxygenase (16). The cavernous smooth muscle produces two types of prostanoids, PGF2 alpha and PGE2, both of which induce relaxation of the cavernous smooth muscle.

The cavernous smooth muscles are tonically contracted in the flaccid state. This allows for decreased arterial blood flow into the penis; therefore, the blood PO_2 in the flaccid state is usually 35 mmHg (17). Upon stimulation, norepinephrine from nerve endings and endothelins and prostaglandin-F from the endothelium activate smooth muscle cells, inositol triphosphate, and diacylglyerol. This causes the release of intracellular calcium, and the opening of calcium channels leads to an influx of calcium from the extracellular space. The influx of calcium initiates a cascade of events including the binding of calcium to calmodulin and the phosphorylation of myosin light chains that allows for smooth muscle contraction.

Pathophysiology of Erectile Dysfunction

Many classification systems have been developed to describe the causes of ED. ED can be classified as due to either specific physiological causes, such as neurogenic, vasculogenic, or endocrine causes, or to psychiatric and psychogenic causes. Other causes include trauma and certain medications. Other classifications of ED have focused on disease states, such as diabetes, prostate disorders, respiratory disorders, and hypogonadism. In this section we present both classification systems to describe the causes of ED.

Neurogenic ED

It is estimated that 10% to 19% of ED cases are neurogenic in origin (18, 19). Neurogenic ED can be classified as having peripheral and central causes. Peripheral neurogenic ED is secondary to disruption of sensory or autonomic nerve fibers to the penis. Conditions associated with peripheral ED include diabetes and having a history of a radical prostatectomy. ED affects up to 80% of men following radical prostatectomy and is a common concern for these patients (20, 21). Central ED is seen in patients who experience a spinal cord injury. Patients with lesions above the sacral parasympathetic centers maintain reflexogenic erections. Minimal tactile stimulation is needed in these patients to induce an erection. Patients with lesions affecting the sacral parasympathetic centers do not have reflex erections and suffer from significant ED. Reflexogenic erection is preserved in 95% of patients who have complete upper cord lesions, whereas only about 25% of those who have complete lower cord lesions can achieve an erection (22). Other pathological processes associated with neurogenic ED include Parkinson's disease, temporal lobe epilepsy, Alzheimer's disease, Shy-Drager syndrome, and encephalitis. It is thought that Parkinson's disease causes ED by causing an imbalance in the dopaminergic pathway (23).

Vasculogenic ED

Vasculogenic ED can be defined as either arterial insufficiency or veno-occlusive dysfunction, also known as venous leak. In patients with arteriogenic ED, the impaired penile artery perfusion is usually due to an atherosclerotic process. Patients with a history of pelvic or perineal trauma usually suffer from focal stenosis of the common penile or cavernous artery (24).

Many recent studies have linked ED to cardiovascular disease. Both conditions have the same risk factors, such as diabetes, hypercholesterolemia, smoking, obesity, hypertension, and advanced age. Thus, it is not surprising that ED serves as a predictor of a heart attack. In the Prostate Cancer Prevention Trial, over 4,000 men without ED were followed prospectively. Of these men, 57% developed some degree of ED within 5 years. Men with ED had a significantly higher incidence of cardiovascular events. In fact, 11% of men experienced a cardiovascular event within 5 years after developing ED, and about 15% had done so within 7 years (25). Another study by Dr. Montorsi and colleagues found that the prevalence of ED was 49% in men with symptomatic coronary artery disease (CAD). These patients noticed ED on average 39 months before the onset of angina (26). Dr. Montorsi attributed these findings to the arterial diameter theory (27). This theory suggests that smaller arteries are more susceptible to endothelial damage and occlusion than larger arteries. This would explain why patients are much more likely to have ED before CAD, CAD before a stroke, and a stroke before they develop peripheral vascular disease. Thus, ED represents an important new means of identifying those at risk of vascular disease. Patients seeking treatment for ED should promptly undergo an assessment of cardiovascular risk factors.

Venogenic ED is due to inadequate venous occlusion. Patients will often describe their inability to maintain their erections. The etiology of venogenic ED includes degenerative changes or trauma to the tunica albuginea that results in inadequate compression of the subtunical and emissary veins. Furthermore, structural changes to the fibroelastic properties of the cavernous smooth muscle, trabeculae, and endothelium may result in venous leak. Increased collagen deposition and decreased elastic fibers in the penile sinusoids are seen in many conditions such as hypercholesterolemia, penile injury, diabetes, and aging (28, 29). The loss of cavernous smooth muscle content is a significant predictor of venous leak. In fact, Sattar and colleagues found that the cavernous tissue of normal potent patients stained more strongly for antidesmin and antiactin than did tissue from patients with venous leak (38.5% and 45.2% vs. 27.4% and 34.2%, respectively) (30). Another cause of venogenic ED is insufficient smooth muscle relaxation, which results in insufficient compression of the subtunical venules. Finally, venogenic ED may be caused by venous shunts, such as those acquired after treatment for priapism (31).

Endocrine Causes

The most common endocrinopathy associated with ED is hypogonadism. Other endocrinopathies associated with ED include hyperprolactinemia and hypothyroidism. Both of these disease states are associated with decreased serum testosterone levels, which in turn contribute to ED.

Androgens and Erectile Function

Androgen deprivation is thought to hinder erectile function through four major mechanisms: impairment of NOS release, altered phosphodiesterase type 5 (PDE5) expression and activity, impaired cavernosal nerve function, and contribution to veno-occlusive disease in the penis.

Animal studies have demonstrated that androgens regulate the expression of NOS isoforms in the corpora cavernosa (32–34). A study by Traish and colleagues demonstrated that castration of adult male rats decreased the activity of penile neural and endothelial NOS, and this was associated with a reduction in erectile response to electrical stimulation of the cavernosal nerve. NO-mediated relaxation of vascular smooth muscle and the cavernosal trabeculae have also been shown to be androgen-dependent (35).

Androgens help maintain innervation of penile tissue. Schirar demonstrated that androgen receptors were present in approximately 40% of neurons in the major pelvic ganglion innervating the corpora cavernosa of the rat penis (36). Giuliano and colleagues have suggested that androgens enhance cavernosal nerve function by acting peripherally in the spinal cord (37). Syme and colleagues studied 45 male Sprague-Dawley rats that underwent bilateral cavernous nerve neurotomy, followed by unilateral nerve graft using the genitofemoral nerve (38). Rats were then randomized to castrate, intact, and testosterone-treated arms. The investigators found that castration resulted in a decreased erectile response to electrostimulation following nerve grafting, while testosterone replacement resulted in a return of erectile response similar to that in intact animals. These studies suggest that androgens may have an effect on cavernosal nerve preservation and function.

Androgen deprivation may be a major contributing factor in veno-occlusive disease through four potential mechanisms: a reduction in trabecular smooth muscle content, changes in fibroelastic properties of the tunica albuginea, increased subtunical fat deposition, and increased deposition of smooth muscle connective tissue. Bhasin and colleagues demonstrated in animal studies that androgens promote the commitment of pluripotent stem cells into a muscle lineage and inhibit their differentiation into adipocytes (39). Thus, lack of androgens can lead to accumulation of adipocytes in the subtunical region of the corpora cavernosa, which in turn can result in an inability of the cavernosal smooth muscle to compress the subtunical venules. Traish and colleagues have demonstrated that androgen deprivation leads to a decrease in cavernosal smooth muscle and decreased intercavernosal pressures after cavernosal nerve stimulation (35).

Finally, studies suggest that androgen deprivation leads to increased corporal smooth muscle collagen deposition by (1) reducing paracrine growth factors (i.e, vascular endothelial growth factor, fibroblast growth factor, and insulin-like growth factor), (2) upregulation of connective tissue proteins (i.e, connective tissue growth factor and transforming growth factor beta 1), and (3) downregulation of metalloproteinases (40). All of these factors contribute to an increase in collagen deposition in the corporal smooth muscle and are thought to contribute to venous leak.

Psychogenic ED

Psychogenic causes of ED stem from the disruption of the balance in excitatory and inhibitory signals that the spinal erection centers receive from the hypothalamus, brainstem, and cerebral cortex. Excessive inhibitory signals to the spinal erection centers will result in ED. Likewise, an abnormally high sympathetic outflow can override an erection due to increased penile smooth muscle contraction. Nocturnal penile tumescence testing can be used to diagnose psychogenic ED. Men able to obtain nocturnal erections are more likely to be suffering from psychogenic ED than organic ED.

Trauma and Medications

Trauma, or iatrogenic trauma, has also been associated with ED. Long-distance cycling is a risk factor for vasculogenic and neurogenic ED due to the chronic trauma in the perineum (41, 42). ED affects up to 80% of men following RP and is a common concern for these patients, as noted above (20, 21). Anywhere from 15% to 100% of men who undergo an abdominal perineal resection and up to 49% of men who undergo an external sphincterotomy will develop ED (43, 44).

Numerous medications have been associated with ED. Antihypertensive medications frequently associated with ED are beta-adrenoceptor antagonists, such as atenolol, and diuretics, such as hydrochlorothiazide (45–47). In contrast, angiotensin-converting enzyme (ACE) inhibitors have not been shown to affect erectile function; in fact, angiotensin II receptor antagonists have been shown to improve ED in men more than placebos (45, 47). Other medications associated with ED include anti-androgens, antidepressants, and psychotropic medications (such as antipsychotic and anxiolytic drugs).

Prostate Disorders and ED

Over the past decade there has been increased interest in studying the relationship between lower urinary tract symptoms (LUTS) and ED. LUTS commonly occur with benign prostatic hypertrophy because of bladder outlet obstruction. Numerous studies support a positive correlation between the degree of LUTS and the degree of ED (48–51). Depending on the degree of LUTS, the relative risk of ED is 1.8 to 7.5 (48–51). This means that moderate to severe LUTS are the second greatest risk factor for ED, after the patient's age. Although a causal relationship has been found between ED and LUTS, the pathophysiology and our understanding of this relationship are not entirely clear. Four plausible theories are proposed to explain the link (50): (1) prostate and penile ischemia, (2) increased Rho-kinase activation/endothelin activity, (3) effect of autonomic hyperactivity on LUTS, prostate growth, and ED, and (4) decreased levels of NO activity in the prostate and penile smooth muscle. While all four of these explanations individually, or in combination, are possible, there is much stronger evidence to support the latter two theories.

There is evidence to suggest that decreased levels of NO are present in the prostate and cavernosal smooth muscle in patients with LUTS and ED (50). Preliminary studies using phosphodiesterase 5 inhibitors show improvement in LUTS. Mulhall and colleagues reported improvements in LUTS in patients treated with sildenafil for their ED, with a mean improvement in the International Prostate Symptom Score (IPSS) of 4.6 points (p = .013) (52). Similarly, Sairam and colleagues showed that a cohort of patients had improved LUTS scores after treatment with sildenafil alone (53). Finally, Adolfsson and colleagues demonstrated that sildenafil may block proliferation of cultured prostatic smooth muscle cells (54).

Respiratory Diseases and ED

Chronic obstructive pulmonary disease (COPD) is a common chronic disease in men. Dyspnea and hypoxemia diminish a patient's functional capacity and can lead to ED. The prevalence of ED in patients with respiratory disease has been reported as high as 75% (55). Several investigators have demonstrated that worsening of pulmonary function test results correlates with the severity of a man's ED (55).

There are many causes of ED in patients with COPD. Disruption of the hypothalamic-pituitary-gonadal axis has been reported in patients with COPD (56). Reversal of hypoxemia with long-term oxygen treatment has been shown to be effective in improving potency (57).

Obstructive sleep apnea (OSA) is also a common chronic respiratory disease. OSA is found in up to 10% of men over 40 years old (58). Recurrent intermittent hypoxemia and transient increases in sympathetic tone during apneic episodes result in an increased risk of daytime somnolence, hypertension, and ischemic cardiovascular events. ED has also been found to be associated with OSA, but more commonly in the most severe cases of OSA (59). Causes for ED in these patients include hypoxemia-driven neural damage, microvascular endothelial damage from increased sympathetic tone and hypertension, low gonadotropin secretion, and psychosocial abnormalities, including daytime somnolence and depressed mood (60–62).

Diabetes and Metabolic Syndrome

Over 47 million people have metabolic syndrome in the United States (63). Metabolic syndrome is a combination of medical disorders that increase an individual's risk for CAD and diabetes. Components of the syndrome include abdominal obesity, atherogenic dyslipidemia, hypertension, insulin resistance, prothrombotic states, and pro-inflammatory states (64). Correlation between metabolic syndrome and ED is well established and mirrors the association of CAD or diabetes with the syndrome. The reported prevalence of ED in patients with metabolic syndrome falls between 26.7% and virtually 100%, and this prevalence increases as the number of components of the metabolic syndrome increases (65, 66).

ED is common in men with diabetes, with a prevalence of 28% to 83% (67). Men with diabetes are three times more likely to have ED than those without diabetes. Furthermore, ED has been found to be age-dependent and is accelerated in age-matched diabetic men. ED affects those with diabetes an average of 10 to 15 years earlier than the general population regardless of insulin-dependence status (68, 69). The onset of ED typically is gradual, with decreased rigidity being the initial manifestation. The resultant premature atherosclerotic changes and microangiopathy seen with diabetes may significantly alter the penile vasculature, but central and peripheral neuropathies have an important role.

In diabetic men ED may be multifactorial in origin, involving possible vascular, neurological, and endocrinological components (70). Conditions that have been shown to be independently associated with ED, such as renal failure, hypertension, and chronic liver disease, often coexist with diabetes. While these comorbid conditions make the association between ED and diabetes coincidental, there is convincing evidence of a correlation between glycemic control in diabetic men and degree of erectile function. One study compared mean hemoglobin A1c (HbA_{1c}) levels in potent diabetic men with those in impotent ones (71). The mean HbA_{1c} levels in the potent group were significantly lower than those in their impotent counterparts. Another study in men with ED found that as the mean HbA_{1c} increased, the mean erectile function score decreased (International Index of Erectile Function questionnaire). They concluded that as glycemic control worsened, potency also declined (72). Furthermore, McCulloch and colleagues found that poor glycemic control was predictive of subsequent development of ED in a 5-year longitudinal study of 466 diabetic men (73). Strict control of blood glucose levels may delay the onset of ED.

Conclusion

Penile tumescence and detumescence are complex physiological phenomena that are controlled by numerous peripheral and central neurotransmitters, hormones, and motor and/or sensory stimulation. It is important to understand the physiology of erections and the pathophysiology of ED so we can better manage and prevent it.

References

1. Lue TF. Erectile dysfunction. *N Engl J Med* 2000;342:1802.

2. Lue TF, Takamura T, Schmidt RA, et al. Hemodynamics of erection in the monkey. *J Urol* 1983;130:1237.

3. Bosch RJ, Benard F, Aboseif SR, et al. Penile detumescence: characterization of three phases. *J Urol* 1991;146: 867.

4. Sachs BD, Meisel RL. The physiology of male sexual behavior. In Knobil E, Neill JD, LL Ewing, Greenwald GS, Market CL, Pfaff DW, eds. *The Physiology of Reproduction*. New York: Raven Press, 1988:1393–1423.

5. Saenz de Tejada I, Goldstein I, Azadzoi K, et al. Impaired neurogenic and endothelium-mediated relaxation of penile smooth muscle from diabetic men with impotence. *N Engl J Med* 1989;320:1025.

6. Andersson KE, Wagner G. Physiology of penile erection. *Physiol Rev* 1995;75:191.

7. Veronneau-Longueville F, Rampin O, Freund-Mercier MJ, et al. Oxytocinergic innervation of autonomic nuclei controlling penile erection in the rat. *Neuroscience* 1999;93:1437.

8. Tang Y, Rampin O, Calas A, et al. Oxytocinergic and serotonergic innervation of identified lumbosacral nuclei controlling penile erection in the male rat. *Neuroscience* 1998;82:241.

9. Melis MR, Spano MS, Succu S, et al. The oxytocin antagonist d(CH2)5Tyr(Me)2-Orn8-vasotocin reduces non-contact penile erections in male rats. *Neurosci Lett* 1999;265:171.

10. Burnett AL, Lowenstein CJ, Bredt DS, et al. Nitric oxide: a physiologic mediator of penile erection. *Science* 1991;257:401.

11. Saenz de Tejada I, Kim N, Lagan I, et al. Regulation of adrenergic activity in penile corpus cavernosum. *J Urol* 1989;142:1117.

12. Hedlund H, Andersson KE. Comparison of the responses to drugs acting on adrenoreceptors and muscarinic receptors in human isolated corpus cavernosum and cavernous artery. *J Auton Pharmacol* 1985;5:81.

13. Saenz de Tejada I, Moroukian P, Tessier J, et al. Trabecular smooth muscle modulates the capacitor function of the penis. Studies on a rabbit model. *Am J Physiol* 1991;260:H1590.

14. Hatzichristou DG, Saenz de Tejada I, Kupferman S, et al. In vivo assessment of trabecular smooth muscle tone, its application in pharmaco-cavernosometry and analysis of intracavernous pressure determinants. *J Urol* 1995;153:1126.

15. Fournier GR Jr, Juenemann KP, Lue TF, et al. Mechanisms of venous occlusion during canine penile erection: an anatomic demonstration. *J Urol* 1987;137:163.

16. Hata AN, Breyer RM. Pharmacology and signaling of prostaglandin receptors: multiple roles in inflammation and immune modulation. *Pharmacol Ther* 2004;103:147.

17. Sattar AA, Salpigides G, Vanderhaeghen JJ, et al. Cavernous oxygen tension and smooth muscle fibers: relation and function. *J Urol* 1995;154:1736.

18. Aboseif S, Shinohara K, Borirakchanyavat S, et al. The effect of cryosurgical ablation of the prostate on erectile function. *Br J Urol* 1997;80:918.

19. Abicht JH. Testing the autonomic system. In Jonas U, Thon WF, Stief CG, eds. *Erectile Dysfunction*. Berlin: Springer Verlag, 1991:187–194.

20. Rabbani F, Stapleton AM, Kattan MW, et al. Factors predicting recovery of erections after radical prostatectomy. *J Urol* 2000;164:1929.

21. Meuleman EJ, Mulders PF. Erectile function after radical prostatectomy: a review. *Eur Urol* 2003;43:95.

22. Eardley I, Kirby RS. Neurogenic impotence. In Kirby RS, Carson CC, Webster GD, eds. *Impotence: diagnosis and management of male erectile dysfunction*. Oxford, England: Butterworth-Heinemann, 1991:227–231.

23. Wermuth L, Stenager E. Sexual aspects of Parkinson's disease. *Semin Neurol* 1992;12:125.

24. Levine FJ, Greenfield AJ, Goldstein I. Arteriographically determined occlusive disease within the hypogastric-cavernous bed in impotent patients following blunt perineal and pelvic trauma. *J Urol* 1990;144:1147.

25. Thompson IM, Tangen CM, Goodman PJ, et al. Erectile dysfunction and subsequent cardiovascular disease. *JAMA* 2005;294:2996.

26. Montorsi F, Briganti A, Salonia A, et al. Erectile dysfunction prevalence, time of onset and association with risk factors in 300 consecutive patients with acute chest pain and angiographically documented coronary artery disease. *Eur Urol* 2003;44:360.

27. Montorsi P, Ravagnani PM, Galli S, et al. The artery size hypothesis: a macrovascular link between erectile dysfunction and coronary artery disease. *Am J Cardiol* 2005;96:19M.

28. Hayashi K, Takamizawa K, Nakamura T, et al. Effects of elastase on the stiffness and elastic properties of arterial walls in cholesterol-fed rabbits. *Atherosclerosis* 1987;66:259.

29. Cerami A, Vlassara H, Brownlee M. Glucose and aging. *Sci Am* 1987;256:90.

30. Sattar AA, Haot J, Schulman CC, et al. Comparison of anti-desmin and anti-actin staining for the computerized analysis of cavernous smooth muscle density. *Br J Urol* 1996;77:266.

31. Dean RC, Lue TF. Physiology of penile erection and pathophysiology of erectile dysfunction. *Urol Clin North Am* 2005;32:379.

32. Lugg J, Ng C, Rajfer J, et al. Cavernosal nerve stimulation in the rat reverses castration-induced decrease in penile NOS activity. *Am J Physiol* 1996;271:E354.

33. Garban H, Marquez D, Cai L, et al. Restoration of normal adult penile erectile response in aged rats by long-term treatment with androgens. *Biol Reprod* 1995;53:1365.

34. Baba K, Yajima M, Carrier S, et al. Delayed testosterone replacement restores nitric oxide synthase-containing nerve fibres and the erectile response in rat penis. *BJU Int* 2000;85:953.

35. Traish AM, Munarriz R, O'Connell L, et al. Effects of medical or surgical castration on erectile function in an animal model. *J Androl* 2003;24:381.

36. Schirar A, Chang C, Rousseau JP. Localization of androgen receptor in nitric oxide synthase- and vasoactive intestinal peptide-containing neurons of the major pelvic ganglion innervating the rat penis. *J Neuroendocrinol* 1997;9:141.

37. Giuliano F, Rampin O, Schirar A, et al. Autonomic control of penile erection: modulation by testosterone in the rat. *J Neuroendocrinol* 1993;5:677.

38. Syme DB, Corcoran NM, Bouchier-Hayes DM, et al. The effect of androgen status on the structural and functional success of cavernous nerve grafting in an experimental rat model. *J Urol* 2007;177:390.

39. Bhasin S, Taylor WE, Singh R, et al. The mechanisms of androgen effects on body composition: mesenchymal pluripotent cell as the target of androgen action. *J Gerontol A Biol Sci Med Sci* 2003;58:M1103.

40. Traish AM, Guay AT. Are androgens critical for penile erections in humans? Examining the clinical and preclinical evidence. *J Sex Med* 2006;3:382.

41. Ricchiuti VS, Haas CA, Seftel AD, et al. Pudendal nerve injury associated with avid bicycling. *J Urol* 1999;162:2099.

42. Andersen KV, Bovim G. Impotence and nerve entrapment in long distance amateur cyclists. *Acta Neurol Scand* 1997;95:233.

43. Yeager E S, Van Heerden J A. Sexual dysfunction following proctocolectomy and abdominoperineal resection. *Ann Surg* 1980;191:169.

44. McDermott DW, Bates RJ, Heney NM, et al. Erectile impotence as complication of direct vision cold knife urethrotomy. *Urology* 1981;18:467.

45. Srilatha B, Adaikan PG, Arulkumaran S, et al. Sexual dysfunction related to antihypertensive agents: results from the animal model. *Int J Impot Res* 1999;11:107.

46. Simonsen U, Prieto D, Hernandez M, et al. Adrenoceptor-mediated regulation of the contractility in horse penile resistance arteries. *J Vasc Res* 1997;34:90.

47. Doumas M, Tsakiris A, Douma S, et al. Factors affecting the increased prevalence of erectile dysfunction in Greek hypertensive compared with normotensive subjects. *J Androl* 2006;27:469.

48. Seftel AD, Rosen RC, Rosenberg MT, et al. Benign prostatic hyperplasia evaluation, treatment and association with sexual dysfunction: practice patterns according to physician specialty. *Int J Clin Pract* 2008;62:614.

49. Rosen RC, Wei JT, Althof SE, et al. Association of sexual dysfunction with lower urinary tract symptoms of BPH and BPH medical therapies: results from the BPH Registry. *Urology* 2009;73:562.

50. McVary K. Lower urinary tract symptoms and sexual dysfunction: epidemiology and pathophysiology. *BJU Int* 2006;97(Suppl 2):23.

51. Braun MH, Sommer F, Haupt G, et al. Lower urinary tract symptoms and erectile dysfunction: co-morbidity or typical "aging male" symptoms? Results of the Cologne Male Survey. *Eur Urol* 2003;44:588.

52. Mulhall JP, Guhring P, Parker M, et al. Assessment of the impact of sildenafil citrate on lower urinary tract symptoms in men with erectile dysfunction. *J Sex Med* 2006;3:662.

53. Sairam K, Kulinskaya E, McNicholas TA, et al. Sildenafil influences lower urinary tract symptoms. *BJU Int* 2002;90:836.

54. Adolfsson PI, Ahlstrand C, Varenhorst E, et al. Lysophosphatidic acid stimulates proliferation of cultured smooth muscle cells from human BPH tissue: sildenafil and papaverin generate inhibition. *Prostate* 2002;51:50.

55. Koseoglu N, Koseoglu H, Ceylan E, et al. Erectile dysfunction prevalence and sexual function status in patients with chronic obstructive pulmonary disease. *J Urol* 2005;174:249.

56. Semple PD, Beastall GH, Brown TM, et al. Sex hormone suppression and sexual impotence in hypoxic pulmonary fibrosis. *Thorax* 1984;39:46.

57. Aasebo U, Gyltnes A, Bremnes RM, et al. Reversal of sexual impotence in male patients with chronic obstructive pulmonary disease and hypoxemia with long-term oxygen therapy. *J Steroid Biochem Mol Biol* 1993;46:799.

58. Lavie P. Incidence of sleep apnea in a presumably healthy working population: a significant relationship with excessive daytime sleepiness. *Sleep* 1983;6:312.

59. Margel D, Cohen M, Livne PM, et al. Severe, but not mild, obstructive sleep apnea syndrome is associated with erectile dysfunction. *Urology* 2004;63:545.

60. Mayer P, Dematteis M, Pepin JL, et al. Peripheral neuropathy in sleep apnea. A tissue marker of the severity of nocturnal desaturation. *Am J Respir Crit Care Med* 1999;159:213.

61. Fanfulla F, Malaguti S, Montagna T, et al. Erectile dysfunction in men with obstructive sleep apnea: an early sign of nerve involvement. *Sleep* 2000;23:775.

62. Akashiba T, Kawahara S, Akahoshi T, et al. Relationship between quality of life and mood or depression in patients with severe obstructive sleep apnea syndrome. *Chest* 2002;122:861.

63. Ford ES. Prevalence of the metabolic syndrome defined by the International Diabetes Federation among adults in the U.S. *Diabetes Care* 2005;28:2745.

64. Ford ES. Leukocyte count, erythrocyte sedimentation rate, and diabetes incidence in a national sample of US adults. *Am J Epidemiol* 2002;155:57.

65. Esposito K, Giugliano F, Martedi E, et al. High proportions of erectile dysfunction in men with the metabolic syndrome. *Diabetes Care* 2005;28:1201.

66. Esposito K, Giugliano D. Obesity, the metabolic syndrome, and sexual dysfunction. *Int J Impot Res* 2005;17:391.

67. Klein R, Klein BE, Lee KE, et al. Prevalence of self-reported erectile dysfunction in people with long-term IDDM. *Diabetes Care* 1996;19:135.

68. Feldman HA, Goldstein I, Hatzichristou DG, et al. Construction of a surrogate variable for impotence in the Massachusetts Male Aging Study. *J Clin Epidemiol* 1994;47:457.

69. Feldman HA, Goldstein I, Hatzichristou D, et al. Impotence and its medical and psychosocial correlates: results of the Massachusetts Male Aging Study. *J Urol* 1994;151:54.

70. Korenman SG. New insights into erectile dysfunction: a practical approach. *Am J Med* 1998;105:135.

71. Bemelmans BL, Meuleman EJ, Doesburg WH, et al. Erectile dysfunction in diabetic men: the neurological factor revisited. *J Urol* 1994;151:884.

72. Romeo JH, Seftel AD, Madhun ZT, et al. Sexual function in men with diabetes type 2: association with glycemic control. *J Urol* 2000;163:788.

73. McCulloch DK, Young RJ, Prescott RJ, et al. The natural history of impotence in diabetic men. *Diabetologia* 1984;26:437.

Chapter 3

Causes and Risk Factors for Erectile Dysfunction

Robert A. Kloner, Thorsten Reffelmann, and
Ernst R. Schwarz

Vascular Causes of ED

While the causes of ED are varied, research since the late 1980s has revealed an important association between vascular disorders and ED, with significant implications for the treatment of ED as well as for risk assessment in cardiovascular medicine: a disproportionately high prevalence of cardiovascular risk factors and manifest cardiovascular disease was demonstrated in men with ED. In addition, a surprisingly high proportion of men with cardiovascular disease have comorbid ED (1–4).

In the longitudinal, population-based Massachusetts Male Aging Study, heart disease, diabetes mellitus, and hypertension were identified as major risk factors for incident ED over 8.8 years of follow-up in men aged 40 to 69 years (5). A prevalence of 44% for hypertension, 23% for diabetes mellitus, 16% for smoking, 79% for obesity, and 74% for elevated low-density lipoprotein cholesterol levels (>120 mg/dL) was reported among men with ED in another investigation (2).

Atherosclerosis, Peripheral Artery Disease, Coronary Artery Disease, and ED

A generalized vascular process involving atherosclerosis and endothelial dysfunction appears to be the basis for many forms of ED, commonly termed vascular-type ED. In 30 patients with ED, flow-dependent vasodilation of the brachial artery, measured as the change in brachial artery diameters before and after inflation of a cuff around the wrist, was strongly associated with first symptoms of ED prior to manifestation of atherosclerotic disease in comparison with age-matched controls (6). Endothelial dysfunction, characterized by reduced vasodilation as a consequence of endothelium-derived factors, which is mainly due to reduced availability or functioning of nitric oxide, appears to be the link between cardiovascular disease and vascular-type ED (7, 8).

Endothelial dysfunction can be regarded as an early stage in the atherosclerotic disease process; thus, the association of atherosclerotic disease with ED is very suggestive. In hypertensive men with ED, a significantly higher carotid intima-media thickness and carotid-femoral pulse wave velocity, along with impaired flow-mediated vasodilation, was demonstrated in comparison with hypertensive men without ED (9). Peak systolic velocity in the penile arterial system (Doppler ultrasound) is considered a correlate of vascular-type ED, and recently the cavernous artery intima-media thickness was introduced as a useful parameter for corroborating the hypothesis that ED may indeed be of vascular origin (10).

Atherosclerotic stenoses and occlusions of the arteries that bring blood to the penile vasculature may also be a reason for compromised sexual function. For instance, the Leriche syndrome, stenoses of the common and internal iliac arteries and pudendal arteries, may contribute to ED. Due to the generalized nature of atherosclerosis and vascular dysfunction, however, revascularization procedures will not always restore sexual function (11, 12).

Similarly, because atherosclerosis tends to be a generalized process, associations between ED and the ankle–brachial index, a parameter indicating peripheral artery disease of the lower extremities, were relatively close (13, 14). Moreover, small-vessel disease of the lower extremities, measured as toe–brachial index, was shown to be associated with the severity of ED (15).

Most importantly, a similar association exists with coronary artery disease: coronary endothelial function, assessed by intracoronary Doppler-derived flow velocity in response to acetylcholine, was closely related to ED (16). Patients with ED had a high incidence of myocardial ischemia, in particular in type 2 diabetics (17, 18). Approximately 75% of patients with silent coronary artery disease have some degree of ED (19). In diabetic patients with silent coronary artery disease, ED significantly predicts cardiovascular events and death, as shown in 291 diabetics with silent coronary artery disease documented by angiography over a mean follow-up of 47.2 months (20). The association of ED with cardiovascular events was confirmed in a substudy of the ONTARGET-TRANSCEND trial (1,549 high-risk patients with coronary, peripheral, cerebrovascular arterial disease or diabetes with end-organ damage, randomized to receive ramipril, telmisartan, or both) (21). Without differences among the specific treatment groups, ED significantly predicted all-cause deaths (hazard ratio [95% confidence interval]: 1.84 [1.21–2.81]), cardiovascular deaths (1.93 [1.13–3.29]), and myocardial infarction (2.02 [1.13–3.58]) over a median follow-up of 56 months.

Diabetes Mellitus and ED

Whether the association of diabetes mellitus with ED is termed vascular-type ED or is summarized under endocrinological disorders is academic. However, in addition to vascular dysfunction, neuropathic alterations may contribute to ED in type 1 and type 2 diabetes mellitus. Among patients with diabetes mellitus, ED was identified as a predictor of silent coronary artery disease apart from traditional risk factors (20). For diabetic patients a strong association between glycemic control and the prevalence of ED is well established (22, 23). In a cross-sectional study investigating men aged 62.0 ± 12.3 years with a mean glycated hemoglobin of 8.1 ± 1.9%, glycated hemoglobin and the presence of peripheral neuropathy were independent predictors of ED (22). Nonetheless, reversal of ED after intensified treatment of diabetes mellitus has not been convincingly shown (24). Most probably, interventions must be initiated at a very early stage of the disease to be effective. Intensified glucose control, along with treatment of concomitant risk factors, may also prevent deterioration of sexual function, even if an improvement cannot be achieved.

Arterial Hypertension and ED

Arterial hypertension is another cardiovascular risk factor that has a strong relation to ED (25–28). Among men seeking medical care for any reason, 61% of those with arterial hypertension, 67% of those with diabetes mellitus, and 78% of those with hypertension and diabetes reported some degree of ED (28). In patients with a non-dipping pattern by ambulatory blood pressure monitoring, the prevalence of ED appears to be slightly higher than in hypertensive patients with a dipping pattern (29). A recent systematic investigation revealed progressive worsening of ED with higher blood pressure levels. Interestingly, in the initial stages of peripheral arterial disease, assessed by the ankle–brachial index, hypertensive men tended to have less severe grades of ED than normotensive patients (30). Nonetheless, arterial hypertension should be treated to achieve target blood pressure levels as a primary or secondary preventive measure. This may be particularly true for patients with ED because they are at high risk for a cardiovascular event. It appears reasonable to assume that effective lowering of blood pressure also attenuates the vascular process responsible for ED, even if there is no scientific proof that sexual function improves with effective blood pressure control. Many drugs, including antihypertensives, may worsen erectile function to some degree as a drug-specific side effect (27). Table 3.1 presents a list of drug classes used in hypertension therapy that have ED as a potential side effect. Thiazide diuretic drugs and slightly less frequently beta-blocking agents are the antihypertensives with the highest incidence of ED; angiotensin-receptor blockers and the beta-blocking agent with direct vasodilating properties, nebivolol, may actually decrease symptoms of ED.

Table 3.1 Drug Classes Used in the Treatment of Arterial Hypertension and Their Effect on Erectile Function (31)	
Thiazide diuretics, such as hydrochlorothiazide	Relatively high incidence of ED; may be attenuated by a low-calorie diet
Beta-blocking agent (exception: nebivolol)	Relatively high incidence of ED; when used as an antianginal drug, consider replacement by ivabradine or ranolazine
Calcium antagonist	Relatively low incidence of ED; sometimes induction of prolactinemia, which may decrease sexual function
Loop diuretics	Low incidence of ED, but sometimes not first choice for antihypertensive therapy
Angiotensin-converting enzyme inhibitor	Low rate of ED; may be replaced by angiotensin-receptor blockers
Angiotensin-receptor blockers	May slightly improve sexual function (preliminary data)
Aldosterone-receptor antagonists	Limited information; in theory eplerenone could be advantageous in comparison with spironolactone (Aldactone)
Renin inhibitor	Limited information
Centrally acting antihypertensives	Limited information

Heart Failure and ED

Heart failure is the number-one entity in cardiovascular medicine in the Western world and in particular in the United States that has increasing prevalence, in part secondary to the increased longevity with older patients surviving acute cardiovascular events. Since heart failure is associated with endothelial dysfunction, it is not surprising that vascular areas dependent on intact endothelial function might be affected as well. In fact, there is a substantial lack of data in the heart failure population with regard to sexual (dys-)function. Risk factors that are common and contribute to the development of cardiovascular diseases such as coronary artery disease, which might lead to ischemic cardiomyopathy and heart failure, are also considered risk factors for the development of ED (32, 33). In particular diabetes mellitus, hypertension, dyslipidemia, and smoking are associated both with cardiovascular disorders and ED. In addition, use of medications such as thiazide diuretics, digoxin, and some beta-blockers is believed to worsen or sometimes even to cause sexual dysfunction in men (34). Furthermore, left ventricular dysfunction in advanced stages leads to reduced cardiac capacity, reduced overall physical functioning, and decreased exercise tolerance and deconditioning secondary to generalized and muscle weakness. All of these factors might contribute additionally to the development and worsening of ED in men. Heart failure patients experience decreased libido and frequency of coitus, ED, negative changes in sexual performance, and a general dissatisfaction related to their sexual function. A questionnaire surveillance study among 100 patients with chronic heart failure in a stable hemodynamic condition showed that 87% of women were diagnosed with female sexual dysfunction and 84% of men had ED (35). An observational, cross-sectional study of heart failure patients with an ejection fraction of 40% or less in two sites in Louisiana and Florida (99 African Americans, 52 Hispanics, 178 Caucasians) revealed a high prevalence of ED among the different ethnic groups (African Americans 95%, Hispanics 85%, Caucasians 92%) (36). Similarly, a relative high prevalence of male sexual dysfunction of 62% has been found in a lower-middle-income country with a developing economy in Eastern Europe, with a prevalence of ED of 61.7% (37).

Sexual activity requires, in the orgasmic phase, an oxygen consumption (VO(2)) between 10 and 14 mL/min/kg. Patients with heart failure usually have diminished oxygen consumption. A recent study showed that none of the heart failure patients with a peak VO(2) of less than 10 mL/min/kg had normal sexual function, while 10 of the 29 patients with peak VO(2) between 10 and 14 mL/min/kg had normal or slightly reduced sexual performance (38). Of interest, a recent study showed a trend toward an increased risk of death but no significant correlation between ED and mortality among heart failure patients (39).

In summary, there is a very high prevalence of ED in men with chronic heart failure. Data on sexual dysfunction in women are sparse. The causes of sexual dysfunction in heart failure are multifactorial and include reduced cardiac capacity, endothelial dysfunction, hormonal imbalances, as well as medication side effects, among other causes (Table 3.2) (40–42). Treatment is often geared toward improving the underlying cardiac condition with the relatively safe use of PDE-5 inhibitors in stable heart failure patients (43, 44). The clinical significance of ED in heart failure patients, its impact on quality of life, and the treatment options are oftentimes not well recognized by patients as well as health care providers.

Table 3.2 Causes/Contributing Factors for ED in Patients with Chronic Heart Failure

Arterial insufficiency
Endothelial dysfunction
Reduced cardiac capacity
Deconditioning, reduced exercise tolerance
Medication side effects (digoxin, diuretics, beta-blockers, aldosterone antagonists, antidepressants)
Fear of cardiac events, performance anxiety, depression
Hormonal imbalances and circulating vasoconstrictors (low androgens, high endothelins)

Other Causes of ED

Causes of ED other than vascular ones should be considered in every patient, and a detailed history and physical examination should be performed to rule in or out these potential causes. Apart from neurological, urological, and anatomical disorders and conditions following spinal cord injury or prostate surgery, many medical diseases are commonly associated with some degree of ED. Among others, the endocrine disorders associated with ED comprise hypogonadism, thyroid disorders, and hyperprolactinemia (also drug-induced). Sickle cell disease and renal and liver dysfunction should also be considered. Specific urological conditions must be explored. Table 3.3 presents an overview of diseases and drugs to be considered in a patient with ED.

Table 3.3 Causes and Risk Factors to be considered when Evaluating Patients Presenting with ED (31)

Cardiovascular risk factors
Arterial hypertension, diabetes mellitus, smoking, dyslipidemia, family history of atherosclerotic disease, sedentary lifestyle, obesity, left ventricular dysfunction, heart failure
Urological disease conditions
Prostate disease or prostate surgery, lower urinary tract infection, Peyronie's disease, priapism, genital trauma
Neurological diseases
Spinal cord injury/paraplegia, cerebrovascular insult, peripheral neuropathy (e.g., diabetic neuropathy)
Medical disorders
Kidney dysfunction and hemodialysis, liver dysfunction, endocrine disorders (hypogonadism, hyperprolactinemia, hypo- and hyperthyroidism), sickle cell disease, leukemia
Psychological factors
Major depression, anxiety disorders, etc.
Medication and drugs side effects

References

1. Virag R, Bouilly P, Frydman D. Is impotence an arterial disorder? A study of arterial risk factors in 440 impotent men. *Lancet* 1985;1(8422):181–184.

2. Walczak MK, Lokhandwala N, Hodge MB, Guay AT. Prevalence of cardiovascular risk factors in erectile dysfunction. *J Gend Specif Med* 2002;5(6):19–24.

3. Blumentals WA, Gomez-Caminero A, Joo S, Vanappagari V. Should erectile dysfunction be considered as a marker for acute myocardial infarction? Results from a retrospective cohort study. *Int J Impot Res* 2004;16(4):350–353.

4. Seftel AD, Sun P, Swinkle R. The prevalence of hypertension, hyperlipidemia, diabetes mellitus and depression in men with erectile dysfunction. *J Urol* 2004;171(6 pt 1):2341–2345.

5. Johannes CB, Araujo AB, Feldman HA, Derby CA, Kleinman KP, McKinlay JB. Incidence of erectile dysfunction in men 40 to 69 years old: longitudinal results from the Massachusetts Male Aging Study. *J Urol* 2000;163(2):460–463.

6. Kaiser DR, Billups K, Mason C, Wetterling R, Lundberg JL, Bank AJ. Impaired brachial artery endothelium-dependent and -independent vasodilation in men with erectile dysfunction and no other clinical cardiovascular disease. *J Am Coll Cardiol* 2004;43(2):179–184.

7. Solomon H, Man JW, Jackson G. Erectile dysfunction and the cardiovascular patient: endothelial dysfunction is the common denominator. *Heart* 2003;9(3):251–253.

8. Schwartz BG, Economides C, Mayeda GS, Burstein S, Kloner RA. The endothelial cell in health and disease: its function, dysfunction, measurement and therapy. *Int J Impot Res* 2010;22(2):77–90.

9. Vlachopoulos C, Aznaouridis K, Iokeimidis N, et al. Arterial function and intima-media thickness in hypertensive patients with erectile dysfunction. *J Hypertens* 2008;26(9):1829–1836.

10. Caretta N, Palego P, Schipilliti M, Ferlin A, Di Mambro A, Foresta C. Cavernous artery intima-media thickness: a new parameter in the diagnosis of vascular erectile dysfunction. *J Sex Med* 2009;6(4):1117–1126.

11. Rogers JH, Karimi H, Kao J, et al. Internal pudendal artery stenoses and erectile dysfunction: correlation with angiographic coronary artery disease. *Catheter Cardiovasc Interv* 2010;76(6):882–887.

12. Rao DS, Donatucci CF. Vasculogenic impotence. Arterial and venous surgery. *Urol Clin North Am* 2001;28(2):309–319.

13. Polonsky TS, Taillon LA, Sheth H, Min JK, Archer SL, Ward RP. The association between erectile dysfunction and peripheral arterial disease as determined by screening ankle-brachial index testing. *Atherosclerosis* 2009;207(2):440–444.

14. Blumentals WA, Gomez-Caminero A, Joo S, Vannappagari V. Is erectile dysfunction predictive of peripheral vascular disease? *Aging Male* 2003;6(4):217–221.

15. Chai SJ, Barrett-Connor E, Gamst A. Small-vessel lower extremity arterial disease and erectile dysfunction: The Rancho Bernardo study. *Atherosclerosis* 2009;203(2):620–625.

16. Elesber AA, Solomon H, Lennon RJ, et al. Coronary endothelial dysfunction is associated with erectile dysfunction and elevated asymmetric diethylarginine in patients with early atherosclerosis. *Eur Heart J* 2006;27(7):824–831.

17. O'Kane PD, Jackson G. Erectile dysfunction: Is there silent obstructive coronary disease? *Int J Clin Pract* 2001;55(3):219–220.

18. Gazzaruso C, Giordanetti D, De Amid E, et al. Relationship between erectile dysfunction and silent myocardial ischemia in apparently uncomplicated type 2 diabetic patients. *Circulation* 2004;110(1):22–26.

19. Kloner RA, Mullin SH, Shook T, et al. Erectile dysfunction in the cardiac patient: how common and should we treat? *J Urol* 2003;170(2pt2):S46–S50.

20. Gazzaruso C, Solerte SB, Pujia A, et al. Erectile dysfunction as a predictor of cardiovascular events and death in diabetic patients with angiographically proven asymptomatic coronary artery disease: a potential protective role for statins and 5-phosphodiesterase inhibitors. *J Am Coll Cardiol* 2008;51(21):2040–2044.

21. Böhm M, Baumhäkel M, Teo K, et al. Erectile dysfunction predicts cardiovascular events in high-risk patients receiving telmisartan, ramipril, or both. *Circulation* 2010;121(12):1439–1446.

22. Romeo JH, Seftel AD, Madhum ZT, Aron DC. Sexual function in men with diabetes type 2: association with glycemic control. *J Urol* 2000;163(3):788–91.

23. Awad H, Salem A, Gadalla A, El Wafa NA, Mohamed OA. Erectile function in men with diabetes type 2: correlation with glycemic control. *Int J Impot Res* 2010;22(1):36–39.

24. Yaman O, Akand M, Gursoy A, Erdogan MF, Anafarta K. The effect of diabetes mellitus treatment and good glycemic control on the erectile function in men with diabetes mellitus-induced erectile dysfunction: a pilot study. *J Sex Med* 2006;3(2):344–348.

25. Bansal S. Sexual dysfunction in hypertensive men: a critical review of the literature. *Hypertension* 1988;12(1):1–10.

26. Kloner RA. Hypertension as a risk factor for erectile dysfunction: implications for sildenafil use. *J Clin Hypertens* 2000;2(1):33–36.

27. Burchardt M, Burchardt T, Baer L, et al. Hypertension is associated with severe erectile dysfunction. *J Urol* 2000;164(4):1188–1191.

28. Giuliano FA, Leriche A, Jaudinot EO, de Gendre AS. Prevalence of erectile dysfunction among 7689 patients with diabetes or hypertension, or both. *Urology* 2004;64(6):1196–1201.

29. Erden I, Ozhan H, Ordu S, Yalcin S, Caglar O, Kayikci A. The effect of non-dipper pattern of hypertension on erectile dysfunction. *Blood Press* 2010;19(4):249–253.

30. Spessoto LC, Cordeiro JA, de Godoy JM. Effect of systemic arterial blood pressure on erectile dysfunction in the initial stages of chronic arterial insufficiency. *BJU Int* 2010;106(11):1723–1725.

31. Reffelmann T, Kloner RA. Sexual function in hypertensive patients receiving treatment. *Vasc Health Risk Manag* 2006;2(4):447–455.

32. Lue TF. Erectile dysfunction. *N Engl J Med* 2000;342:1802–1813.

33. Schwarz ER, Rodriguez J. Sex and the heart. *Int J Impot Res* 2005;17:S4-S6.

34. Schwarz ER. Rastogi S, Kapur V, Sulemanjee N, Rodriguez JJ. Erectile dysfunction in heart failure patients. *J Am Coll Cardiol* 2006;19:1111–1119.

35. Schwarz ER, Kapur V, Bionat S, Rastogi S, Gupta R, Rosanio S. The prevalence and clinical relevance of sexual dysfunction in women and men with chronic heart failure. *Int J Impot Res* 2008;20:85–91.

36. Herbert K, Lopez B, Castellano J, Palacio A, Tamari L, Arcemen LM. The prevalence of erectile dysfunction in heart failure patients by race and ethnicity. *Int J Impot Res* 2008;20:507–511.

37. Hebert K, Anand J, Trahan P, et al. Prevalence of erectile dysfunction in systolic heart failure patients in a developing country: Tbilisi, Georgia, Eastern Europe. *J Sex Med* 2010;7:3991–3996.

38. Apostolo A, Vignati C, Brusoni D, et al. Erectile dysfunction in heart failure: correlation with severity, exercise performance, comorbidities, and heart failure treatment. *J Sex Med* 2009;6:2795–2805.

39. Hebert K, Lopez B, Macedo FY, Gomes CR, Urena J, Arcement LM. Peripheral vascular disease and erectile dysfunction as predictors of mortality in heart failure patients. *J Sex Med* 2009;6:1999–2007.

40. Schwarz ER, Rastogi S, Kapur V, Sulemanjee N, Rodriguez JJ. Erectile dysfunction in heart failure patients. *J Am Coll Cardiol* 2006;48:1111–1119.

41. Rastogi S, Rodriguez JJ, Kapur V, Schwarz ER. Why do patients with heart failure suffer from erectile dysfunction? A critical review and suggestions on how to approach this problem. *Int J Impot Res* 2005;17(Suppl 1):S25–36.

42. Kapur V, Schwarz ER. The relationship between erectile dysfunction and cardiovascular disease. Part I: pathophysiology and mechanisms. *Rev Cardiovasc Med* 2007;8:214–219.

43. Kapur V, Chien CV, Fuess JE, Schwarz ER. The relationship between erectile dysfunction and cardiovascular disease. Part II: The role of PDE-5 inhibition in sexual dysfunction and cardiovascular disease. *Rev Cardiovasc Med* 2008;9:187–195.

44. Vural A, Agacdiken A, Celikyurt U, et al. Effect of cardiac resynchronization therapy on libido and erectile dysfunction. *Clin Cardiol* 2011 Jun 2 [E-pub].

Chapter 4

Diagnostic Evaluation of Erectile Dysfunction

Raymond M. Bernal

Introduction

The question of whether a patient has erectile dysfunction (ED) is easy to answer. As defined by the National Institutes of Health Consensus Development Panel on Impotence, ED is the recurrent inability to attain and/ or maintain a penile erection sufficient for intercourse (1). This definition was modified at the International Consultation on Sexual Medicine (ICSM) in 2004, which established time intervals by which "recurrent inability" could be defined. Thenceforth, the diagnosis of ED required the persistence of symptoms for a minimum of 3 months, but would allow for diagnosis at a shorter interval if the ED were secondary to traumatic or surgical reasons (2). In general, the diagnosis of ED relies on patient self-report, with objective testing serving as an adjunct measure.

Thus, in most cases, it is not a question of whether a patient has a functional erectile problem, as this can be easily established by the above criteria; it is a question of why.

Historically, many believed that impotence was due to psychological problems. Masters and Johnson believed that more than 90% of impotence cases were due to psychogenic causes (3). With the introduction of vascular and prosthetic surgical techniques in the 1970s to address the organic physiological causes of ED, testing evolved to delineate which patients would be best served by surgery. Nocturnal penile tumescence testing, brachial penile indices, cavernosometry, internal pudendal arteriography, and color duplex Doppler ultrasonography were some of the tools developed to evaluate patients with ED. With a better understanding of ED pathophysiology, not only was there a shift in diagnoses from psychogenic to organic ED, but different subclasses of organic ED were realized. Vascular, neurological, and endocrine abnormalities were increasingly implicated in the development of ED.

In the 1980s, with the varied tests and therapies to treat ED, as well as the extensive standard evaluation of all patients with ED, clinicians realized the value of limiting diagnostic tests to those that would influence the ultimate treatment choice. The diagnosis and treatment strategy became "goal-directed," taking into account patients' ultimate treatment preferences (4). In 1998, sildenafil was introduced to treat ED. With the availability of a safe, highly effective, noninvasive, and device-independent means to treat ED, diagnostic testing to identify patients who might benefit from surgery became less important. For men with ED, a pill could be offered, and if it worked, rigorous workup became unnecessary. Combined with health care mandates to minimize unnecessary testing, routine invasive investigations were abandoned.

Nevertheless, finding the root causes to ED may help guide treatment if initial empirical oral therapies fail. It is hoped that elucidating these will result in treatment plans that are more specific and efficacious. Because the pathophysiology of ED is complex and the disorder can involve myriad pathologies, determining its contributing factors can set the framework for a multidisciplinary ED solution.

With an understanding that rigorous testing is not always indicated, a framework for the diagnostic evaluation of ED is presented. Recent guidelines for evaluation have been established by the American Urological Association, the European Association of Urology, and the International Society of Sexual Medicine. Notably, the 2009 International Consultation in Sexual Medicine Committee Consensus Report established general principles of patient evaluation by which sexual dysfunction should be evaluated. In summary, a detailed sexual history, medical history, and psychosocial history are mandatory, a focused physical examination and laboratory tests are highly recommended, and specialized testing and referral are recommended if the results of these evaluations indicate further evaluation (5).

Patient History

The patient interview should focus on identifying ED risk factors and characterizing the nature of the problem. Initiating the discussion of ED should be done in a private setting, and the clinician should address the interview in a sensitive fashion (6). The patient's unique personal and cultural backgrounds should be acknowledged in the interview (7). Clinicians should be nonjudgmental and empathetic to make the patient feel comfortable in disclosing and discussing potentially sensitive and embarrassing information.

Using validated patient-reported questionnaires to screen for and assess the severity of ED can help to initiate a discussion. These forms can be completed prior to the visit, and review of the patients' responses can lead into a conversation. There are several validated questionnaires available. In general, they are used as diagnostic aids to supplement the clinical history and evaluation in the diagnosis of ED and can serve as instruments to assess the patient's ED over time.

The most common clinically used questionnaire to evaluate ED is the Sexual Health Inventory for Men (SHIM), a five-item abridged version of the International Index of Erectile Function (IIEF) (8). It has been translated and validated in several languages. The following questions are used to reflect the patient's experience over the preceding 6 months:

1. How did you rate your confidence that you could get and keep an erection?
2. When you had erections with sexual stimulation, how often were your erections hard enough for penetration?

3. During sexual intercourse, how often were you able to maintain your erection after you had penetrated your partner?
4. During sexual intercourse, how difficult was it to maintain your erection to completion of intercourse?
5. When you attempted sexual intercourse, how often was it satisfactory to you?

Questions are scored from zero or one to five, and the severity of the patient's ED is suggested depending on the total summed score: severe (score of 1–7), moderate (score of 8–11), mild to moderate (score of 12–16), mild (score of 17–21), and no ED (score of 22–25). Providers should ask about the patient's opportunity for sexual activity, as the SHIM was not designed to assess men without sexual partners (9). Patients' sexual partners can be insightful during the interview, and a validated six-item questionnaire, the Female Assessment of Male Erectile Dysfunction Detection Scale (FAME), was developed to aid in the diagnosis of ED by the female partner (10). Other questionnaires have been validated and can capture other useful data regarding sexual health. For example, the unabridged IIEF questionnaire, although longer, captures additional data regarding sexual desire and orgasm.

A thorough sexual history should include the onset and duration of ED, as well as the severity of dysfunction and possible medical or psychosocial risk factors. Previous treatment regimens should be asked about to determine the patient's responses and any side effects. The patient should be questioned about the presence of any erectile activity in the morning or during sleep. Assessment of erections during masturbation or with certain partners may provide insight into ED that may be exacerbated or primarily due to performance anxiety or other psychogenic issues. The nature of erectile firmness during sexual activity can be asked about, and a patient-reported Erection Hardness Score can be determined and followed over time. This can range from 0 to 4, determined by the following criteria: 0, penis does not enlarge; 1, penis is larger but not hard; 2, penis is hard but not hard enough to penetrate; 3, penis is hard enough to penetrate but not completely hard; and 4, penis is completely hard and fully rigid (11). Asking about other sexual dysfunction, such as the presence of ejaculatory dysfunction or low sexual desire, may hint at endocrine or relationship problems and is important in assessing overall sexual function. The health of the partner should be asked about, as insecurity about sexual safety with partners in poor health can evoke anxiety.

A complete medical history should be reviewed, and risk factors for ED, including hypertension, dyslipidemia, peripheral vascular disease, coronary artery disease, diabetes, autonomic dysfunction, spinal cord injury, chronic kidney disease, psychiatric disorders, pituitary disease, thyroid disorders, hypogonadism, Peyronie's disease, priapism, pelvic radiation, and penile trauma, should be noted. A thorough surgical history should also be asked about, with special attention to pelvic surgery, genital surgery, neurological surgery, and aortoiliac vascular surgery.

A complete review of systems should be performed to look for symptoms in other systems that may uncover reasons for ED. Headaches and double vision could indicate a pituitary disorder, claudication may indicate penile vascular disease, neuropathies or paresthesias might indicate autonomic or somatic nerve dysfunction, and polydipsia with polyuria may help to diagnose diabetes. Recreational tobacco, alcohol, and illicit drug use should be reviewed, as all can contribute to ED. Hobbies such as prolonged cycling should also be noted. Patients should be asked about their exercise tolerance to estimate their cardiovascular status, as this is important in determining their ability to have sexual activity without risking a coronary event (12).

Medications should be reviewed, with special attention to medications that can cause ED such as beta-blockers, thiazides, clonidine, selective serotonin reuptake inhibitors, tricyclic antidepressants, antiseizure medications, antihistamines, H_2 blockers, opiates, methadone, muscle relaxants, nonsteroidal anti-inflammatory agents, and antiandrogens. Many medications have been associated with ED, and each should be checked as a possible cause. Importantly, medications that may be contraindicated for use with phosphodiesterase inhibitors, such as nitrates, and those that should be separated by time during administration, such as alpha-blockers, should be noted.

Physical Examination

A directed physical examination may suggest medical problems contributing to ED. Manifestations of endocrine dysfunction, vascular disease, neurological pathology, trauma, and Peyronie's disease can be revealed during the examination. Recommendations from the 2009 ICSM state that physical examination is highly recommended when evaluating men with sexual dysfunction, but not always necessary (7). This is because often the physical examination cannot secure the diagnosis of ED. Nonetheless, the physical examination may uncover significant medical disease that may be modulated to improve erectile function. As such, careful attention to vital signs and physical examination is important.

Elevated blood pressure readings may suggest chronic hypertension and atherosclerosis. An elevated Body Mass Index, as determined by measuring height and weight, can be associated with diabetes, lipid abnormalities, and hypogonadism. Gynecomastia, soft and small testicles, regression of facial and body hair, loss of muscle mass, and increased abdominal fat can be characteristic of low testosterone or free testosterone levels. Double vision or loss of peripheral vision may suggest a pituitary disorder. Scars potentially indicate direct trauma to sexual organs or to the nerves and vessels that supply them. Penile plaques and curvature are indicative of Peyronie's disease. Genital sensation, anal tone, and the bulbocavernosus reflex may be diminished in neurological disorders. Weak or absent pulses and associated skin changes may suggest peripheral vascular disease.

Laboratory Tests

The 2009 ICSM recommendations also point out that routine laboratory evaluations are highly recommended but not always necessary (7). Similar to the physical examination, discovery of abnormal laboratory values may uncover abnormalities that can predispose patients to ED. Tests for pituitary adenomas, thyroid disorders, hypogonadism, diabetes, and hyperlipidemia may uncover treatable causes of ED.

Initial laboratory tests to consider include a fasting glucose, lipid panel, and total testosterone. As fasting levels are ideal for the former tests, and a morning draw is ideal for the latter, these should all be drawn in the early morning. If the total testosterone level is low, a repeat testosterone assessment can be obtained to confirm the low value. A free testosterone level may also be obtained, but this may be costly. An alternative is to also determine the amount of sex hormone binding globulin present, and to calculate a free testosterone level from a widely accessible online formula: http://www.issam.ch/freetesto. htm (13). Measuring the prostate specific antigen level may be useful if considering testosterone replacement therapy.

Optional tests include serum luteinizing hormone and prolactin levels. These may be investigated if the testosterone level is low to detect endocrine axis abnormalities. Also optional is screening for thyroid dysfunction, which if detected and treated may help improve testosterone production and erectile function.

Diagnostic Testing

Tests that can be used to evaluate ED range from noninvasive nocturnal penile tumescence testing to invasive arterial angiography (14). Routine specialized diagnostic testing has lost favor because well-tolerated oral therapies for ED have become widely available and evaluation to accurately determine the cause of ED has become less relevant, given this treatment success. Nonetheless, specialized testing is justifiable when determining the etiology of ED is desired, and when characterization may guide treatment selection. These tests can be especially helpful after conservative treatment has failed and surgery is planned.

Testing for Psychogenic ED

The observation of normal erections in patients complaining of ED has been used to suggest psychogenic causes. These can be in response to eroticism or during periods of rapid eye movement sleep. In patients without neurovascular risk factors for ED and with a history suggesting psychogenic ED, nocturnal penile tumescence testing can be offered. This test may not be useful in patients with mood disorders, nightmares, fatigue, sleep deprivation, apnea, and substance abuse, as sleep erections can be adversely affected (15). Erections are documented by utilizing the RigiScan device, which uses two loops that are placed around the penis and a recording computer. Essentially, these loops tighten periodically to measure outward radial force at the base and toward the tip of the penis, and can determine periods of erection and estimate penile rigidity. Over a sleep period of 8 hours, recordings of three to six erections lasting an average of 10 to 15 minutes, with base rigidities of 55% to 60% and tip rigidity of 50%, indicate what many consider normal erections (16). Psychogenic ED can be diagnosed in patients with suggestive histories and normal erections during this study (17). If erections are abnormal, a three-night test is conducted for confirmation, and further diagnostic testing can be offered to characterize the organic dysfunction with the previous caveats noted.

Testing for Vascular ED

Several tests have been developed to uncover vascular pathologies contributing to ED. Each requires complete cavernous smooth muscle relaxation to maximize penile blood flow, usually accomplished by intracorporal vasoactive medication injection and erotic or self-stimulation (18). Simple observation of a firm erection after intracorporal vasoactive injection implies that the penile venous occlusion mechanism is functioning during erection. Poor erectile response, however, may signify either poor venous occlusion or suboptimal arterial inflow (19). The addition of duplex ultrasonography is useful in characterizing the nature of vasculogenic dysfunction as secondary to arterial insufficiency, veno-occlusive dysfunction, or mixed disease.

Duplex ultrasonography following intracavernosal injection was popularized in the mid-1980s (20). This technology can be performed in the office setting, and recent guidelines have been published (21). Based on Doppler signals, penile arterial inflow can be directly measured, and venous outflow can be indirectly determined. Both cavernous arteries are examined at the base of the penis at various time intervals after injection. Peak systolic velocities are measured to assess for arterial insufficiency, while end-diastolic velocities are measured to assess for corporal veno-occlusive dysfunction. Calculation of a resistive index can help determine mixed pathologies. Using high-resolution ultrasound, anatomical abnormalities can be detected, such as vascular anomalies from trauma and calcifications or fibrosis associated with Peyronie's disease (22). Should veno-occlusive dysfunction be detected, and the patient desire further workup to determine whether surgical intervention can remedy the problem, the patient can be offered dynamic infusion cavernosometry and cavernosography (DICC) to determine the nature of the venous leak (23).

In DICC, quantification of venous leak can be determined by infusing saline into the cavernosal bodies to achieve intracavernosal pressures equal to mean arterial pressure. The flow rate at which erection is sustained is measured. It is imperative that cavernosal smooth muscle is maximally relaxed during this evaluation. The location of leak can be determined by using contrast to perform the cavernosography. Given the invasiveness of this test, it is usually reserved for young patients with ED, or those with a history of Peyronie's disease or penile trauma who may have distinct areas of venous leak amenable to vein ligation (24).

Selective pudendal arteriography can be offered to young men who are suspected of having a distinct area of narrowing in their penile inflow circulation. Men with a history of ED following penile or perineal trauma are the usual candidates. The pudendal artery is accessed via an endovascular approach, and contrast is injected to assess the entire penile arterial circulation. If treatable stenosis is detected, penile revascularization can be offered (25).

Testing for Neurogenic and Myogenic ED

Currently, there are no widely accepted definitive tests to diagnose neurogenic ED secondary to autonomic nerve damage or cavernosal smooth muscle pathology. Corpus cavernosum electromyography (ccEMG), which is similar in concept to electrocardiography monitoring, is a noninvasive study involving skin electrodes on the penis to measure sympathetic activity of the cavernosal smooth muscle cells. It was developed in the 1980s and has been able to detect smooth muscle degeneration and autonomic neuropathy in patients with ED. However, it is not widely available, and more testing has to be done to determine precise ccEMG patterns for different pathologies and to establish parameters of normalcy (26).

New Methods

There are many diagnostic vascular tests in development. Gadolinium-enhanced magnetic resonance angiography has been used as a noninvasive means of assessing the penile vasculature, including both arterial (27) and venous (28) systems. Other diagnostic tests that are being explored for greater clinical application include near-infrared spectrophotometry, radioisotopic penography, tissue oximetry, laser Doppler flowmetry, quantification of circulating endothelial progenitor cells, and general vascular testing as indicators of penile vessel atherosclerosis or endothelial dysfunction (14).

Conclusion

A self-reported complaint of ED can secure the diagnosis. A detailed history supplemented with validated questionnaires, a limited physical examination, and pertinent laboratory tests are indicated during the initial diagnostic workup. By doing so, ED risk factors and medical comorbidities may be uncovered and treated, and quantification of treatment responses can be determined by follow-up questionnaires. Keeping with the contemporary patient-centered and goal-directed approach to ED, further diagnostic workup should be offered in cases of conservative treatment failure when the patient is considering invasive therapies such as vascular or prosthetic surgery, or if the patient wishes to understand why he is suffering from ED. With a thorough workup, the delay to appropriate treatment can be minimized. Most importantly, however, is that a thorough diagnostic evaluation may uncover dangerous comorbidities, allow an opportunity to direct positive lifestyle changes, and lead to overall improved health and well-being through appropriate referral and treatment.

References

1. Consensus development conference statement. National Institutes of Health. Impotence. December 7–9, 1992. *Int J Impot Res* 1993;5(4):181–284.

2. Lue TF, Giuliano F, Montorsi F, et al. Summary of the recommendations on sexual dysfunctions in men. *J Sex Med* 2004;1(1):6–23.

3. Masters WH, Johnson V. *Human Sexual Inadequacy*. Boston: Little Brown & Company, 1970.

4. Lue TF. Impotence: a patient's goal-directed approach to treatment. *World J Urol* 1990;8(2):67–74.

5. Montorsi F, Adaikan G, Becher E, et al. Summary of the recommendations on sexual dysfunctions in men. *J Sex Med* 2010;7(11):3572–3588.

6. Rosen RC. Evaluation of the patient with erectile dysfunction: history, question-naires, and physical examination. *Endocrine* 2004;23(2–3):107–111.

7. Hatzichristou D, Rosen RC, Derogatis LR, et al. Recommendations for the clini-cal evaluation of men and women with sexual dysfunction. *J Sex Med* 2010;7(1 Pt 2):337–348.

8. Rosen RC, Cappelleri JC, Smith MD, Lipsky J, Pena BM. Development and evaluation of an abridged, 5-item version of the International Index of Erectile Function (IIEF-5) as a diagnostic tool for erectile dysfunction. *Int J Impot Res* 1999;11(6):319–326.

9. Cappelleri JC, Rosen RC. The Sexual Health Inventory for Men (SHIM): a 5-year review of research and clinical experience. *Int J Impot Res* 2005;17(4):307–319.

10. Rubio-Aurioles E, Sand M, Terrein-Roccatti N, et al. Female Assessment of Male Erectile dysfunction detection scale (FAME): development and validation. *J Sex Med* 2009;6(8):2255–2270.

11. Mulhall JP, Goldstein I, Bushmakin AG, Cappelleri JC, Hvidsten K. Validation of the erection hardness score. *J Sex Med* 2007;4(6):1626–1634.

12. Kostis JB, Jackson G, Rosen R, et al. Sexual dysfunction and cardiac risk (the Second Princeton Consensus Conference). *Am J Cardiol* 2005;96(2):313–321.

13. Vermeulen A, Verdonck L, Kaufman JM. A critical evaluation of simple meth-ods for the estimation of free testosterone in serum. *J Clin Endocrinol Metab* 1999;84(10):3666–3672.

14. Meuleman EJ, Hatzichristou D, Rosen RC, Sadovsky R. Diagnostic tests for male erectile dysfunction revisited. Committee Consensus Report of the International Consultation in Sexual Medicine. *J Sex Med* 2010;7(7):2375–2381.

15. Jannini EA, Granata AM, Hatzimouratidis K, Goldstein I. Use and abuse of RigiScan in the diagnosis of erectile dysfunction. *J Sex Med* 2009;6(7):1820–1829.

16. Guay AT, Heatley GJ, Murray FT. Comparison of results of nocturnal penile tumescence and rigidity in a sleep laboratory versus a portable home monitor. *Urology* 1996;48(6):912–916.

17. Basar MM, Atan A, Tekdogan UY. New concept parameters of RigiScan in differentiation of vascular erectile dysfunction: is it a useful test? *Int J Urol* 2001;8(12):686–691.

18. Meuleman EJ, Diemont WL. Investigation of erectile dysfunction. Diagnostic testing for vascular factors in erectile dysfunction. *Urol Clin North Am* 1995;22(4):803–819.

19. Donatucci CF, Lue TF. The combined intracavernous injection and stimulation test: diagnostic accuracy. *J Urol* 1992;148(1):61–62.

20. Lue TF, Hricak H, Marich KW, Tanagho EA. Vasculogenic impotence evalu-ated by high-resolution ultrasonography and pulsed Doppler spectrum analysis. *Radiology* 1985;155(3):777–781.

21. AIUM practice guideline for the performance of an ultrasound examination in the practice of urology. *J Ultrasound Med* 2012;31(1):133–144.

22. LeRoy TJ, Broderick GA. Doppler blood flow analysis of erectile function: who, when, and how. *Urol Clin North Am* 2011;38(2):147–154.

23. Mulhall JP, Anderson M, Parker M. Congruence between veno-occlusive param-eters during dynamic infusion cavernosometry: assessing the need for caverno-sography. *Int J Impot Res* 2004;16(2):146–149.

24. Vardi Y, Glina S, Mulhall JP, Menchini F, Munarriz R. Cavernosometry: is it a dinosaur? *J Sex Med* 2008;5(4):760–764.

25. Goldstein I, Bastuba M, Lurie A, Lubisich J. Penile revascularization. *J Sex Med* 2008;5(9):2018–2021.

26. Meuleman E, Jiang X, Holsheimer J, Wagner G, Knipscheer B, Wijkstra H. Corpus cavernosum electromyography with revised methodology: an explorative study in patients with erectile dysfunction and men with reported normal erectile function. *J Sex Med* 2007;4(1):191–198.

27. Stehling MK, Liu L, Laub G, Fleischmann K, Rohde U. Gadolinium-enhanced magnetic resonance angiography of the pelvis in patients with erectile impotence. *Magma* 1997;5(3):247–254.

28. Kurbatov DG, Kuznetsky YY, Kitaev SV, Brusensky VA. Magnetic resonance imaging as a potential tool for objective visualization of venous leakage in patients with veno-occlusive erectile dysfunction. *Int J Impot Res* 2008;20(2):192–198.

Chapter 5

Treatment for Erectile Dysfunction

Andrew C. Kramer and Ellen R. Goldmark

Oral Treatment Options: Phosphodiesterase Type 5 Inhibitors

Introduction

Phosphodiesterase type 5 (PDE-5) inhibitors were discovered serendipitously in 1985, when scientists were looking for a compound to lower blood pressure (1). The mechanism of this compound was to potentiate the effects of cGMP and ultimately lower blood pressure through vasodilatation (2). PDE-5 breaks down cGMP and converts it back to the inactive compound GMP. This in turn becomes GTP and via guanylate cyclase is converted back to the active cGMP (3). By inhibiting cGMP's breakdown, the vasodilatory effects of this compound are enhanced and prolonged (2).

In 1989, Pfizer created sildenafil, and clinical trials ensued to examine its efficacy in lowering blood pressure. Despite lackluster results as an antihypertensive agent, patients seemed reluctant to return unused medication at the end of the trial, exposing the drug's unintended effect: it increased erectile function. The class of drugs known as PDE-5 inhibitors was born, and with it came enhanced enthusiasm in discussing, recognizing, and treating erectile dysfunction (ED). Today, three pills with similar mechanisms exist: sildenafil, vardenafil, and tadalafil (4). With many years of successful results from these drugs, as well as a reasonably minimal side-effect profile, these oral erectogenic agents continue to be first-line therapy for organic ED.

PDE-5 Usage

The PDE-5 inhibitors are quite similar in chemical structure and not surprisingly have similar actions. With slight exceptions, these drugs are all intended to be used on demand (5). This implies that they are taken only as needed, in a 30-minute to 1-hour window in anticipation of a sexual encounter. Then these pills provide a substantial period of enhanced genital blood flow and tumescence, only in response to stimulation in the course of the natural erectile response. The pills have rarely induced priapism if taken on their own and as directed (6), and will not create an erection without stimulation or arousal.

The maximal dose of sildenafil is 100 mg, and the highest dose of vardenafil and tadalafil is 20 mg. The side-effect profile and onset of action vary slightly among these medications, but the general theme is similar. For all of these erectogenic pills, the patient takes a pill in anticipation of the sexual encounter on an as-needed basis, with a response created after stimulation. The only situations where one would use daily PDE-5 inhibitor therapy would be the use of the Cialis daily pill, which is made in either 2.5-mg or 5-mg formulations (7), or in the setting of penile rehabilitation.

Penile Rehabilitation

These pills were initially intended to be on-demand medications rather than daily pills. A notable exception to this is in the emerging school of thought surrounding penile rehabilitation. In many practices, patients who undergo a radical prostatectomy will be offered a course of aggressive treatment after surgery to mitigate the loss of potency that tends to occur. In some institutions this includes a vacuum device, intracavernosal injection therapy, and in some cases, daily use of a PDE-5 inhibitor. Data from many institutions have demonstrated that daily use of an erectogenic medication has resulted in earlier recovery of erectile function, and improved potency at earlier time endpoints (8, 9). Given the relatively safe side-effect profile, those who oppose this aggressive therapy point primarily to cost and lack of solid data as reasons not to use daily PDE-5 inhibitors for penile rehabilitation.

Efficacy and Side-Effect Profile

The response in large clinical trials for all of the PDE-5 inhibitors has been positive and robust. Several of the larger studies indicated qualitative improvements in erectile function of 70% to 80%, versus 20% to 30% for placebo (10). These results have been repeatable, leading to relatively widespread acceptance in the medical community. Furthermore, there is no tachyphylaxis with these medications, so while a patient's erectile function may worsen over time, greater drug requirements are not needed to reach the same effect.

The major contraindication of all three PDE-5 inhibitors is the concomitant use of nitroglycerine due to a dangerous drop in blood pressure, and use in patients in whom sexual activity alone would be too great a cardiac stress. Other side effects include headache (13%), flushing (11%), dyspepsia (7%), nasal congestion (4%), and visual changes (3%) (11). These are largely due to systemic vasodilatation, and cross-reactivity to phosphodiesterase in other parts of the body, including the retina (PDE-6) and visceral smooth muscle (PDE-1–5). Despite the side effects, these medications are still very well tolerated. Rarely, cases of nonarteritic ischemic optic neuropathy (NAION) have been reported with the use of sildenafil, resulting in sudden blindness in a small subset of 12 patients. A warning was issued that patients who experience NAION, or who are anxious about possibly developing it while on these medications, should consult an ophthalmologist (12).

Intracavernosal Injectable Therapy

The introduction of the vasoactive agents as a treatment for ED in the 1980s offered an additional method of treatment for ED at a time when few options were available. A self-demonstration of the efficacy of vasoactive agents in inducing erection was given at the American Urological Association (AUA) meeting in 1983 by Brindley, who self-administered phenoxybenzamine (13). Although oral PDE-5 inhibitors have since been introduced, providing an effective, noninvasive means to achieve erection, vasoactive agents, including prostaglandins, papaverine, and alpha-adrenergic antagonists, remain mainstays in ED treatment. Many patients have higher satisfaction with intracavernosal injections (ICI). In a study of 433 men with chronic ED treated with sildenafil citrate, 186 had previously undergone treatment with ICI. Sildenafil was considered inferior to ICI by 43.6% of the men who were given the oral agent (14). Vasoactive agents are best divided into two categories: ICI and transurethral therapy.

Efficacy

ICI therapy is thought to be the most effective treatment for ED not involving surgery. Unfortunately, it is somewhat invasive by nature and has the highest potential for priapism compared to the other treatments for ED (15). According to the 2005 AUA guidelines on ED management, oral PDE-5 inhibitors should be offered as first-line therapy for ED, unless contraindicated. Candidates for ICI therapy include patients who have failed to respond to oral therapy (including diabetic patients and patients with severe vascular disease) and patients who use nitrates or have the potential to do so. Other patients with neurological injury from pelvic surgery, trauma, or radiation may also be ideal candidates for ICI therapy (13). Patients with absolute and relative contraindications for ICI therapy include those who have had a history of priapism with vasoactive drug use or severe penile fibrosis. Patients who use monoamine oxidase inhibitors cannot be given phenylephrine to reverse potential priapism because the combination of these drugs may cause a hypertensive crisis (13).

Method of Use and Mechanism

A health care provider must be present to instruct patients on the proper technique of ICI drug administration to help determine the appropriate dose as well as monitor for priapism (15). Self-injection is performed on the dorsolateral aspect of the penile shaft, away from the dorsal nerve (13). Rigidity is achieved within 2 to 10 minutes as an increase in arterial blood flow results in compression of the subtunical venules between the corpora cavernosa and tunica albuginea (13).

Alprostadil, papaverine, and phentolamine, used together or in combination, are the mainstays of therapy. Alprostadil causes increased cAMP levels through modulation of the enzyme adenyl-cyclase. This increase in the amount of cAMP leads to a decrease in free calcium concentration and subsequent relaxation of the cavernous smooth muscle (16). Papaverine is another agent that can be used in combination with other vasoactive agents to induce erection. It works by causing nonspecific inhibition of phosphodiesterase, causing increased levels of cGMP and cAMP. It also blocks voltage-dependent calcium channels, keeping calcium levels low. Some studies demonstrate an increased risk of priapism (1–6%) and fibrosis (6–12%) compared with other agents (13). Phentolamine, the alpha-adrenergic antagonist, is thought to work through its increase in corporal blood flow to induce erection (13).

The use of PGE-1 with phentolamine and papaverine provides an advantage in that there is a decrease in the volume of each solitary compound, leading to a decrease in cost (16). Bimix (phentolamine and papaverine) and trimix (papaverine, phentolamine, and PGE-1) are available only if a pharmacy offers compounding services. The combination of drugs may increase efficacy or decrease side effects. Usually physician preference guides the initial choice in therapy (15).

Alprostadil can be given through a transurethral route in addition to its intracavernous route. The urethral mucosa's lining of complex columnar cells makes it a surface through which drugs may be absorbed; thus, the compound still increases intracellular concentrations of cAMP (17). Submucosal veins, specifically the circumflex and emissary veins perforating the tunica albuginea, allow transmission of the drug within the corpus spongiosum and corpora cavernosa (18). This will be reviewed in the section below about MUSE.

Vacuum Erection Device

As opposed to the invasive nature of ICI, the vacuum erectile device is a safe, noninvasive method to treat ED. It may be used alone or in combination with injections or PDE-5 inhibitors in the treatment of ED. The theory behind the vacuum erectile device is to use negative pressure to distend the corporal sinusoids and to increase blood inflow to the penis (19). A vacuum constriction device subsequently uses an external constriction ring at the base of the penis to prevent outflow of blood from the corpora cavernosa (19). A vacuum erectile device does not use a constrictive ring. Patients may obtain these devices without a prescription, but the AUA recommends that only vacuum constriction devices containing a vacuum limiter should be used in order to prevent penile injury by preventing high negative pressures (15). Several vacuum erectile devices are on the market and use the same principle, but they vary slightly in their pressure-release valves and the shape/size of their compression rings (20). The patient places a constrictive ring over the open end of the vacuum cylinder and creates negative pressure by hand or a battery-operated pump. It takes between 30 seconds and 7 minutes to produce an erection (19), although patients should be instructed to pump for 1 to 2 minutes and then again for 3 to 4 minutes (20). Once the patient achieves a satisfactory erection, the constriction ring is placed on the base of the penis. The vacuum cylinders are then removed (19).

It is important to tell patients that the constriction ring should not be left on the penis for longer than 30 minutes, as blood gas analysis of the penis has demonstrated ischemia after this length of time (19). Patients should expect that their penis may appear dusky in color and may feel cooler to the touch, with increased size distally (19).

Low patient acceptability limits the use of this treatment method (15). A study by Gilbert and colleagues followed 45 impotent men who failed to respond to ICI. Although 38 men were able to obtain an erection with the vacuum device, only 12 reported satisfactory sexual intercourse (21). However, a study by Cookson and colleagues surveyed 216 patients, of which 115 patients using a vacuum device for a median follow-up of 29 months responded. These patients reported 84% patient and 89% partner satisfaction. Quality of erection was 90% (evaluated for hardness, length, and circumference) (22).

Risks

Patients with fibrosis secondary to priapism, severe proximal leakage, or arterial insufficiency may not achieve an adequate erections with the vacuum device (18). Some patients with poor manual dexterity may have difficulty operating the device. Men with bleeding disorders taking anticoagulants may develop petechiae, although their risk is not increased over that of the general population (19). The most common side effects include penile discomfort, numbness, bruising, and petechiae (19).

Intraurethral Suppository

Another option for ED treatment is using an intraurethral suppository as an erectogenic agent. This is commonly referred to by its trade name, MUSE (Medicated Urethral Suppository for Erection). An applicator is used to deliver a pellet of alprostadil in its 3 × 1-mm form to the distal urethra (18).

A randomized control study involving 1,511 men showed that 50.4% episodes of home administration resulted in successful intercourse (17). Dose-related pain is associated with the drug: during the same trial, penile pain was reported by 35.7% of men, but only 2.4% discontinued use because of it (17). Because of the risk of hypotension and syncope, initial administration must by done in the doctor's office.

Mechanism

MUSE, like the other forms of therapy, works through smooth muscle dilatation and increased blood flow to the corpora (23). The compound alprostadil is administered as a pellet that is roughly the size of a grain of rice, inserted into the urethral meatus with a plastic applicator. Alprostadil is chemically identical to prostaglandin E1, a vasoactive substance naturally found in the human body. This medication was introduced in 1997, at the time offering an acceptable alternative to injectable therapies.

Use and Onset of Action

MUSE typically works within 5 to 10 minutes, and unlike the PDE-5 inhibitors, it will work regardless of the state of patient arousal, since the pellet is inserted directly into the target organ. The goal is to induce an erection that lasts between 30 minutes and an hour, and priapism has rarely been described with this therapy. Intraurethral suppositories can be used in conjunction with a penile implant to engorge the glans (24), because the implant provides rigidity to the corpora cavernosa but leaves the corpus spongiosum soft, absent stimulation. Four strengths of MUSE are available: 125, 250, 500, and 1,000 mcg. Patients are instructed not to use more than 2 units per 24-hour period. Instructions on use include voiding just prior to self-administration, thus lubricating the urethra. Once the pellet is inserted into the urethra, gentle penile massage facilitates absorption.

Risks and Downside

Erectogenic pills, ICI, and penile implants have markedly diminished the use of MUSE. The generally accepted success rate is reported to be between 30% and 40%, with the lower doses reportedly not effective for the average man who presents with ED (25). While this route of administration is less daunting than a cavernosal injection, patients need to be taught to use the applicator and deliver a dose. Complexity of administration has led to significant patient drop-out, as well as pain and discomfort in the penis upon treatment.

Penile Implant Surgery

The first penile implant surgery was described in the early 1970s, but the devices have evolved significantly since the earliest versions (26). The principle behind penile implantation for ED is to introduce a rigid or inflatable structure within the corpora cavernosa, thus providing firmness when the natural erectile response fails to fill the corpora with enough blood for penetration. The available devices vary in complexity and sophistication. Today, there exist the semirigid or malleable penile implant, a two-piece or Ambicore prosthesis, and an inflatable three-piece prosthesis. Broadly, there are two companies that manufacture these devices: Coloplast and American Medical Systems, both based near Minneapolis, Minnesota.

Semirigid and Malleable Devices

The most basic of penile implants is where a noninflatable but pliable rod is inserted into each corpus, providing permanent rigidity (27). The angle of the penis can be altered so it can be either suitable for sexual relations or pointed downward when not in use. This device is simple to use and does not require manual dexterity on the patient's part. There is a low malfunction rate due to fewer operational parts. These have been used outside the realm of sex for spinal cord injury patients requiring condom catheters. In this population, the device makes fitting the condom on the penis easier and more secure. One long-term risk associated primarily with this type of implant is distal erosion, germane to this device specifically because the tips are always hard and give constant pressure to the glans penis (28). Despite the introduction of more complex implants through the years, this device has stood the test of time and is still implanted in certain patients in whom this implant is most appropriate. Some advocate its use in salvage-type procedures. This is when an initial inflatable device becomes infected; in the setting of removal and washout, a semirigid device is introduced. This tendency may be due to less complexity involved in implanting this device, with potentially less risk of infection.

Inflatable Penile Prosthesis

The principle behind an inflatable penile prosthetic device is that it better mimics the action of a healthy penis. These devices have the potential to be soft, when fluid is shifted away from the part of the corporal cylinders in the external phallus, and hard or rigid as fluid is directed into the cylinders of the external phallus. There is an inherent complexity to these inflatable devices because the fluid has to travel between two different spaces: one is some form of reservoir or storage region while the penis is soft, and the other is the cylinders in the external penis when rigid. The patient has control over the flow of fluid within the device by accessing a pump within the scrotum.

An Ambicore or two-piece inflatable prosthesis has a pump, and dual cylinders in the left and right corpora (29). The reservoir in this device is the proximal portion of the corporal cylinders. As the patient depresses the pump, fluid flows from the proximal cylinders into the distal part of the cylinders, and the external phallus becomes rigid. When the patient bends or folds the penis, the fluid is forced back into the proximal penis and detumescence occurs.

A more common implant used today is a three-piece penile prosthesis, which best replicates the actions of the normal penis and gives the patient the best control over his erections. Here, the reservoir is separate from the pump and cylinders and is typically placed into the space of Retzius, or perivesical space (30). This reservoir is in continuity with the pump, connected by tubing. When the patient inflates the device, fluid flows from the reservoir to the cylinders. The pump in these devices has a deflate mechanism whereby fluid leaves the penis, causing compete detumescence, and flows back to the reservoir (30). This type of device is generally constructed with an anti-lockout mechanism built into either the pump or reservoir to prevent unintentional movement of fluid during the Valsalva maneuver. While the most complex and expensive of the aforementioned devices, the three-piece penile prosthesis gives the patient the best control of his erections and over time has given patients high rates of satisfaction. Penile prostheses can be placed either scrotally or infrapubically. Some place the cylinders and pump of the three-piece prosthesis through the scrotum, and place the reservoir with the aid of an inguinal counter-incision.

Risks and Benefits

The risks must be well understood by the patient prior to proceeding with the implantation. Patients should be well informed that this operation is irreversible, in the sense that the corpora must be dilated and filled with the cylinders of a prosthetic device, rendering the normal smooth muscle of the corpora unsalvageable should the device need to be removed. Many physicians refer to penile prosthesis placement as "end-of-the-line therapy" for this reason (31). Another main risk of this procedure is infection of the device, necessitating immediate explantation. Often this infection does not lead to sepsis and systemic bacteremia, but if left untreated, it can make the patient very sick. Another risk in placing any penile implant is injury to the urethra upon placement of the corporal cylinders. Potential risks of inflatable prostheses include injury to the bladder or iliac vessels upon reservoir placement and, down the line, breakage of the device and slight (1–2 cm at most) penile shortening (32). With experience, surgeons can minimize the risks and achieve greater benefits.

The devices have evolved to add sophistication and minimize potential complications. Both brands of three-piece prosthesis are coated with antibiotics (33). The American Medical Systems device is impregnated with antibiotics, and the Coloplast device is coated with antibiotics once dipped in an antibacterial solution at the time of surgery (33). The pumps from both companies' devices have evolved to have one-touch release valves so the patient can easily deflate the devices with one swift motion. The long-term durability of inflatable penile prostheses is well documented, with roughly a 10% breakage rate at 10 years (34). Generally, if a device malfunctions, it can be repaired, or in some cases replaced. While pills are widespread throughout the lay press and medical community, penile prosthetics are placed by a small subset of urologists.

References

1. Ghofrani H, Osterloh I, Grimminger F. Sildenafil: from angina to erectile dysfunction to pulmonary hypertension and beyond. *Nature Reviews Drug Discovery* 2006;5:689–702.

2. Francis SH, Corbin JD. Sildenafil: efficacy, safety, tolerability and mechanism of action in treating erectile dysfunction. *Expert Opin Drug Metab Toxicol* 2005;1:283–293.

3. Murthy KS. Activation of phosphodiesterase 5 and inhibition of guanate cyclase by cGMP dependent protein kinase in smooth muscle. *Biochem J* 2001;360:199–208.

4. Beers MH et al., eds. *The Merck Manual of Medical Information.* 2nd Home Edition. Whitehouse Station, NJ: Merck, 2003.

5. Eardley I. Optimisation of PDE-5 inhibitor therapy in men with erectile dysfunction: converting "non-responders" into "responders." *Eur Urol* 2006;50:31–33.

6. Sur R, Kane CJ. Sildenafil-citrate associated priapism. *Urology* 2000;55:950.

7. McMahon C. Efficacy and safety of daily tadalafil in men with erectile dysfunction previously unresponsive to on-demand tadalafil. *J Sex Med* 2004;1:292–300.

8. Zagaja GP, Mhoon DA, Aikens JE, Brendler CB. Sildenafil in the treatment of erectile dysfunction after radical prostatectomy. *Urology* 2000;56:631–634.

9. Padma-Nathan H, McCullough AR, Giuliano F. Postoperative nightly administration of sildenafil citrate significantly improves the return of normal spontaneous erectile function after bilateral nerve-sparing radical prostatectomy [abstract 1402]. *J Urol* 2003;169.

10. Goldstein I, Lue T, Padma-Nathan H, Rosen R, Steers W, Wicker P. Oral sildenafil in the treatment of erectile dysfunction. *N Engl J Med* 1998;338:1397–1404.

11. Gillies HC, Roblin D, Jackson G. Coronary and systemic haemodynamic effects of sildenafil citrate: From basic science to clinical studies in patients with cardiovascular disease. *Int J Cardiol* 2002;86:131–141.

12. McGwin G, Vaphiades M, Hall T, Owsley C. Non-arteritic anterior ischemic optic neuropathy and the treatment of erectile dysfunction. *Br J Ophthalmol* 2006;90:154–157.

13. Bella A, Brock G. Intracavernous pharmacotherapy for erectile dysfunction. *Endocrine* 2004;23:149–155.

14. McMahon C, Samali R. Efficacy, safety and patient acceptance of sildenafil citrate as treatment for erectile dysfunction. *J Urol* 2000;164:1192–1196.

15. AUA Guidelines on the Management of Erectile Dysfunction: Diagnosis and Treatment Recommendations. AUA Education and Research, Inc., 2005. [Available online].

16. Hartmut P. The rationale for prostaglandin E1 in erectile failure: A survey of worldwide experience. *J Urol* 1998;166:802–815.

17. Padmin-Nathan H, Hellstrom W, Kaiser F. Treatment of men with erectile dysfunction with transurethral alprostadil. *N Engl J Med* 1997;336:1–7.

18. Lue T, Broderick G. Evaluation and nonsurgical management of erectile dysfunction and premature ejaculation. In *Campbell-Walsh Urology*. Elsevier Press, 2011:768–783.

19. Yuan J, Hoang A, Lin H, Dai Y, Wang R. Vacuum therapy in erectile dysfunction: science and clinical evidence. *Int J Impot Res* 2010;22:211–219.

20. Hellstrom W, Montague D, Moncada I. Implants, mechanical devices, and vascular surgery for erectile dysfunction. *J Sex Med* 2010;7:501–523.

21. Gilbert HW, Gingell JC. Vacuum constriction devices: second-line conservative treatment for impotence. *Br J Urol* 1992;70:81–83.

22. Cookson MS, Nadig PW. Long-term results with vacuum constriction device. *J Urol* 1993;149:290–294.

23. Becker K, ed. *Principles and Practice of Endocrinology and Metabolism*. Philadelphia: Lippincott Williams & Wilkins, 2001:957.

24. Benevides M, Carson C. Intraurethral application of alprostadil in patients with failed inflatable penile prosthesis. *J Urol* 2000;163:785–787.

25. McCullough A, Hellstrom W, Wang R, Lepor H, Wagner K, Engel J. Recovery of erectile function after nerve sparing radical prostatectomy and penile rehabilitation with nightly intraurethral alprostadil versus sildenafil citrate. *J Urol* 2010;183:2451.

26. Bettocchi C, Palumbo F, Spilotros M, LucarelliG, Ricapito S, Battaglia M, Selvaggi F, Ditonno P. Penile prosthesis implant: when what and how. *J Mens Health* 2009;6:299–306.

27. Montague D. Experience with semirigid rod and inflatable penile prosthesis. *J Urol* 1983;129: 967–968.

28. Zermann D, Kutzenberger J, Sauerwein D, Schubert J, Loeffler U. Penile prosthesis surgery in neurologically impaired patients: long-term follow-up. *J Urol* 2005;174:1041–1044.

29. Levine L, Estrada C, Mortantaler A. Mechanical reliability and safety of, and patient satisfaction with the Ambicore inflatable penile prosthesis: results of a 2-center study. *J Urol* 2001;166:932–937.

30. Hellstrom W. Three-piece penile prosthesis components (surgical pearls on reservoirs, pumps, and rear tip extenders). *Int J Impot Res* 2003;15:S136-S138.

31. Kramer A, Schweber A. Patient expectations prior to Coloplast Titan penile prosthesis implant predicts postoperative satisfaction. *J Sex Med* 2010;7:2261–2266.

32. Henry G. Management of intraoperative penile implant complications. *Current Sexual Health Reports* 2005;2:64–68.

33. Wilson S, Zumbe J, Henry G, Salem E, Delk J, Cleves M. Infection reduction using antibiotic-coated inflated penile prosthesis. *Urology* 2007;2:337–340.

34. Anastasiadis A, Wilson S, Burkhardt M, Shabsigh R. Long-term outcomes of inflatable penile implants: reliability, patient satisfaction, and complication management. *Curr Opin Urol* 2001;11:619–623.

Chapter 6

Erectile Dysfunction: A Harbinger or Consequence?

Martin M. Miner

Introduction

The presence of erectile dysfunction (ED) has been clearly associated with cardiovascular disease in numerous studies (1–9). In addition, the symptom of ED often precedes the clinical consequences of cardiovascular and cerebrovascular disease.

ED is defined as the inability to reach or maintain erection sufficient for satisfactory sexual performance. Evidence is accumulating in favor of ED as a vascular disorder in the majority of patients. Common risk factors for atherosclerosis are prevalent in patients with ED, and the risk of ED has been related to the number and severity of risk factors themselves (10, 11). In addition, the prevalence of ED is increased in patients with vascular comorbidities such as coronary artery disease (CAD) (12–15), diabetes (11, 16), cerebrovascular disease (17), hypertension, and peripheral arterial disease (18, 19). Finally, ED and cardiovascular disease share a similar pathogenic involvement of the nitric oxide pathway leading to impairment of endothelium-dependent vasodilatation (early phase) and structural vascular abnormalities (late phase) (20–22). Thus, ED may be considered as the clinical manifestation of a vascular disease affecting the penile circulation; likewise, angina pectoris is the clinical manifestation of a vascular disorder affecting coronary circulation. Indeed, in the Montorsi COBRA study of 285 patients with CAD, ED was found to precede CAD by an average of 2 to 3 years (15).

Moreover, there is growing opinion that ED is a marker of increased cardiovascular risk, an index of subclinical coronary disease, and a precursor of cardiovascular events, and a variety of mechanisms have been proposed (15). ED could be a predictor because it leads to depression, which leads in turn to increased cardiac risk. Or men with ED have higher Body Mass Index and greater visceral obesity, or other comorbidities that lead to both ED and CAD (23, 24).

In his landmark 2005 report (4) of over 9,400 men, Thompson and colleagues posed the following questions: "With the high prevalence of erectile dysfunction (ED) in aging men, do pharmacologic, lifestyle, or behavioral interventions that are cardioprotective also reduce or delay onset of erectile dysfunction? Could erectile dysfunction serve as a surrogate measure of treatment efficacy in preventive interventions for cardiac disease?" These questions remain unanswered, but our knowledge is growing significantly.

In Thompson and colleagues' study as part of the Prostate Cancer Prevention Trial, men age 55 years and older who were enrolled in the placebo group (n = 9,457) were evaluated at 3-month intervals for ED and subsequent cardiovascular disease. There were 4,247 men with no ED at study entry; 2,420 developed incident ED (defined as the first report of ED of any grade) over 5 years. Incident (new-onset) ED (adjusted for other cardiovascular risk factors) was associated with a hazard ratio (HR) of 1.25 (95% confidence interval [CI] 1.04–1.53; p = .04) for subsequent cardiovascular events, including myocardial infarction, coronary revascularization, cerebrovascular accident, transient ischemic attack, congestive heart failure, fatal cardiac arrest, or nonfatal cardiac arrhythmia. The adjusted HR was even higher (1.45; 95% CI 1.25–1.69; p < .001) for men with either incident or prevalent ED (i.e., ED at study entry). Therefore, the authors were able to conclude that incident ED had an effect equal to or greater than the effects of family history of myocardial infarction, cigarette smoking, or measures of hyperlipidemia on subsequent cardiovascular events (4).

ED in Diabetics: Does ED Hold Greater Risk in this Population?

Thompson and colleagues' study lent further support to the notion that ED is predominantly a disease of vascular origin, with endothelial cell dysfunction as the unifying link. Investigations in diabetics have also supported this concept and in fact suggest that ED is a predictor of future cardiovascular events in this group. Gazzaruso and colleagues (5) recruited 291 type 2 diabetic men with silent CAD and found that those who developed major adverse cardiac events over the course of approximately 4 years were more likely to have ED (61.2%) than those who did not (36.4%). Through further multivariate analysis, ED remained an important predictor of adverse cardiac events, and although diabetics have a high risk of cardiovascular disease, the risk is even higher in those who develop ED.

Ma and colleagues (6) studied 2,306 diabetic men with no clinical evidence of CAD, of whom 27% had ED. Over the course of approximately 4 years, the incidence of coronary heart disease was greater in men with ED (19.7/1,000 person-years) than in men without ED (9.5/1,000 person-years). After adjustments for other covariates, including age, duration of disease, antihypertensive agents, and albuminuria, ED remained an independent predictor of coronary heart disease (HR 1.58, 95% CI 1.08–2.30, p = .018).

Therefore, because ED and silent CAD are prevalent in the diabetic population, this should move all health care providers in primary care to inquire about sexual function in diabetic patients and aggressively treat cardiovascular risk factors, including dyslipidemia and hypertension. Indeed, the Second Princeton Consensus Panel (24) on sexual activity and cardiac risk published recommendations for individuals with established CAD or suspected CAD related to estimated risk for cardiovascular events, and those individuals of intermediate or indeterminate risk (no overt cardiac symptoms and three or more cardiovascular risk factors, including sedentary lifestyle; moderate stable angina; recent myocardial infarction <6 weeks; NYHA Class II heart failure; prior stroke, transient ischemic attack, or history of peripheral vascular disease) should receive further cardiac evaluation to delineate the presence and severity of coronary disease.

Harbinger or Consequence?

Hackett (25) reviewed the association between ED and its well-known concomitant comorbidities in the context of current knowledge of phosphodiesterase type 5 (PDE-5) inhibitors, to evaluate both safety and efficacy. His analysis revealed compelling evidence for primary care physicians to address underlying cardiovascular health concerns in men presenting with ED. His review suggested that ED is often found in association with other common disorders in primary care, such as diabetes, cardiovascular disease, hypertension, dyslipidemia, obesity, depression, chronic obstructive pulmonary disease, and benign prostatic hypertrophy/lower urinary tract symptoms. He acknowledged the older paradigm that ED can be caused by several of these conditions, but he also highlighted the emerging paradigm that ED may be considered a sentinel marker for occult cardiovascular disease or many of these comorbidities. He further noted that the severity of ED is directly related to vascular risk factors that are associated with endothelial dysfunction, as noted above (22, 26).

It is therefore recommended that physicians screen ED patients for vascular disease, and since ED often coexists with the comorbidities of diabetes (three- to four-fold incidence, according to Hackett), hypertension, or dyslipidemia, screening for ED in the primary care clinician's office should occur with the management of each of these comorbidities (25).

What Does ED Tell Us in the Nondiabetic Population?

What about the nondiabetic population without comorbidities? What does the presence of ED suggest in the lower-risk male population not yet studied to date? To this point, Inman and colleagues (7) biennially screened a random sample of over 1,400 community-dwelling men who had regular sexual partners and no known CAD for the presence of ED over a 10-year period. Men were followed from the fourth screening round (1996) of the Olmsted County Urinary Symptoms and Health Status among Men Study until the first occurrence of an incident cardiac event or the last study visit (December 31, 2005). Men with prevalent ED at study onset were excluded from the analyses. Multivariate proportional hazard regression models were used to assess the association of the covariates of age, diabetes, hypertension, smoking status, and Body Mass Index with ED. Unlike the Thompson and colleagues study or others noted above, the participants in this study were not a highly selected subset of the general male population and greater than 55 years of age, but were more representative of a normal (albeit predominantly Caucasian) group of men. In addition, erectile function of the study participants was assessed by an externally validated questionnaire, the Brief Male Sexual Function Inventory (BMSFI) (27), a self-reported questionnaire comprising 11 items rated on a scale of 0 to 4, with higher scores representing better sexual function.

During the 10-year follow-up period, ED was modeled as a time-dependent covariate that allowed each patient's ED status to change over time, with results stratified by 10-year age periods and adjusted for diabetes, hypertension, smoking status, and Body Mass Index. The baseline prevalence of ED was 2% for 40-year-olds, 6% for 50-year-olds, 17% for 60-year-olds, and 39% for men over the age of 70. New ED developed in 6.4% at 2 years, with increases of approximately 5% in each subsequent 2-year interval over the 10-year period of follow-up. Incident ED was more common in patients with higher cardiovascular risk and older age (7).

Overall, new incident CAD developed in 11% of men over the 10-year follow-up period, with approximately 15% of cases due to myocardial infarction, 79% to angiographic anomalies, and 6% to sudden death. The cumulative incidence of CAD was strongly influenced by patient age. CAD incidence densities per 1,000 person-years for men without ED were 0.94 (age 40–49), 5.09 (age 50–59), 10.72 (age 60–69), and 23.30 (age 70+). For men with ED, the incidence densities for CAD were 48.52 (age 40–49), 27.15 (age 50–59), 23.97 (age 60–69), and 29.63 (age 70+) (7) (Fig. 6.1).

Is ED a Greater Predictor of Cardiovascular Disease in the Younger Man?

The meaning of these findings is most significant. While ED and CAD may be different manifestations of an underlying vascular pathology, when ED occurs

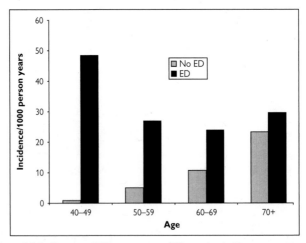

Figure 6.1 Incidence per 1000 person-years of ED associated with coronary artery disease densities (incidence densities in patients with and without ED) (28).

in a younger man (<60), it is associated with a marked increase in the risk of future cardiac events; in older men, it has less prognostic value. While ED had little relationship to the development of incident cardiac events in men aged 70+, it was associated with a nearly 50-fold increase in the 10-year incidence in men 49 years and younger. This raises the possibility of a "window of curability" in which progression of cardiac disease might be slowed or halted by medical intervention. Younger men with ED could provide the ideal populations for future studies of primary cardiovascular risk prevention (8).

In a retrospective study of a cohort of 1,660 men with ED, Chew and colleagues (29) compared a diagnosis of ED to hospital morbidity data and death registrations. They used a standardized incidence rate ratio (SIRR) to describe the incidence of atherosclerotic cardiovascular events subsequent to the manifestation of ED in this cohort to that in the general male population. Men with ED had a statistically significantly higher incidence of atherosclerotic cardiovascular events (SIRR 2.2; 95% CI 1.9–2.4). There were significantly increased incidence rate ratios in all age groups younger than 70 years, but, across all age groups, as age increased, the ED-versus-CV-events relationship diminished ($p < .0001$) (29). Younger age at first manifestation of ED, cigarette smoking, presence of comorbidities, and socioeconomic disadvantage were all associated with higher hazard ratios for subsequent atherosclerotic cardiovascular events (29). These data strongly suggest that ED is a powerful marker for future cardiovascular events and that this may be seen in men as early as their fourth or fifth decades of life.

Why younger than older men? Clearly there is a higher incidence of psychogenic ED in younger men, and the argument can be made that all ED has a psychological component. However, in the younger man with more than one cardiovascular risk factor, his ED and CAD may be different manifestations of an underlying vascular pathology. ED appears to precede symptoms of CAD in patients with a vascular etiology. Montorsi and colleagues (9) suggest that this phenomenon relates to the caliber of the blood vessels. For example, the penile artery has a diameter of 1 to 2 mm, whereas the proximal left anterior descending coronary artery is 3 to 4 mm in diameter. An equal-sized atherosclerotic plaque burden in the smaller penile arteries would more likely compromise flow earlier and cause ED compared to the same amount of plaque in the larger coronary artery causing angina. In another plausible explanation, Inman and others (7) suggest greater impairment in arterial endothelial cell function with age. The repetitive pulsations that the large central arteries are subjected to over their lifespan lead to fatigue and fracture of the elastic lamellae, resulting in increased stiffness (30). Ultimately small arteries such as the pudendal and penile arteries begin to degenerate and end-organ ischemia results. In the younger man with ED, impaired vasodilation of a penile artery is more likely to lead to ED even in the absence of atherosclerotic plaque narrowing the lumen than the same scenario in the coronary arteries leading to symptoms of angina (7).

Hackett (25) goes further to elaborate that in the treatment of ED with PDE-5 inhibitors as a class, and particularly in studies using sildenafil and tadalafil, these agents have been shown to dilate epicardial coronary arteries, improve endothelial dysfunction, and inhibit platelet activation in patients with coronary artery disease (31, 32). The availability of effective, noninvasive treatment methods, which have a significant impact on the quality of life of men with

ED, means that an increase in the diagnosis of ED could benefit a large number of men and their partners and potentially improve the pathology leading to the condition itself.

Although ED is associated with cardiovascular risk factors and atherosclerosis, it is not known whether the presence of ED is predictive of future events in individuals with cardiovascular disease. Bohm and colleagues (32) evaluated whether ED is predictive of mortality and cardiovascular outcomes, and because inhibition of the renin-angiotensin system in high-risk patients reduces cardiovascular events, the investigators wished to establish whether there are protective effects of the pharmacological inhibition of this system. Therefore, the investigators additionally tested the effects on ED of randomized treatments with telmisartan, ramipril, and the combination of the two drugs (ONTARGET), as well as with telmisartan or placebo in patients who were intolerant of angiotensin-converting enzyme inhibitors (TRANSCEND).

In a prespecified substudy, 1,549 patients, 842 of whom had a history of ED at baseline and were slightly older (65.8 years vs. 63.6 years; $p < .0001$), with a higher prevalence of hypertension, stroke/transient ischemic attack, diabetes mellitus, and lower urinary tract symptoms, underwent double-blind randomization, with 400 participants assigned to receive ramipril, 395 telmisartan, and 381 both of them (ONTARGET), as well as 171 participants assigned to receive telmisartan and 202 placebo (TRANSCEND). ED was evaluated at baseline, at 2-year follow-up, and at the penultimate visit before closeout. Clearly, because of the nature of the study population, incident ED or new-onset ED was small. However, either baseline or incident ED was predictive of all-cause death (HR 1.84, 95% CI 1.21–2.81, $p = .005$) and the composite primary outcome (HR 1.42, 95% CI 1.04–1.94, $p = .029$), which consisted of cardiovascular death (HR 1.93, 95% CI 1.13–3.29, $p = .016$), myocardial infarction (HR 2.02, 95% CI 1.13–3.58, $p = .017$), hospitalization for heart failure (HR 1.2, 95% CI 0.64–2.26, $p = .563$), and stroke (HR 1.1, 95% CI 0.64–1.9, $p = .742$). The study medications did not influence the course or development of ED (32).

ED is a potent predictor of all-cause death and the composite of cardiovascular death, myocardial infarction, stroke, and heart failure in men with cardiovascular disease. Trial treatment with either telmisartan or ramipril did not significantly improve or worsen ED (32). This is a bit surprising, given these agents' beneficial effects on endothelial cell function.

Whether ED is only a risk marker or may even be considered a "CAD risk equivalent" (an independent risk factor) is not yet fully clarified, yet there is evidence to consider all men with ED younger than 60 years of age at risk for cardiovascular disease until proven otherwise (33, 34). However, given the high prevalence of ED in the middle-aged population, a systematic cardiologic screening would not be cost-effective. Therefore, it is crucial to identify ED patients at high risk for occult CAD, acute coronary events, or both. The task for the clinician is to identify those patients with ED who may be at intermediate or high risk for subsequent cardiovascular disease (33). A reasonable first step is to estimate, through one of several risk assessment office-based approaches, the subject's own relative and absolute risk of a cardiovascular event (usually in the following 10 years).

Novel Biomarkers or Surrogates to Clarify Cardiovascular Risk in the ED Patient

Risk stratification requires measurement tools of cardiovascular disease risk. These tools must be valid in the population of men with ED as opposed to the general male population. Cardiac biomarkers are measurement tests that help predict cardiac risk (35). Traditional measurements of cardiovascular risk utilize the lipid panel, blood sugar, and blood pressure, but these may be inadequate in the young man with ED, given the high rate of cardiovascular events that occur despite aggressive risk-factor modification in terms of lowering LDL cholesterol. A post hoc analysis of the recent Treating to New Targets (TNT) study found that even with aggressive reductions in LDL cholesterol, low HDL levels and elevated triglyceride levels remained associated with increased coronary risk and subsequent cardiovascular events (36). If one accepts that ED precedes cardiovascular disease, then identifying and stratifying cardiometabolic risk in the younger ED patient is vital. More sensitive markers are needed to pick up early evidence of increased cardiovascular disease risk in this specific population of men.

Nontraditional biomarkers may include anthropomorphic measurements such as waist circumference, Body Mass Index, and other measures of visceral obesity. Erectile function has been negatively associated with these measures (37). Imaging markers include coronary artery calcification scoring as measured by electron-beam computed tomography, or carotid intima-media thickness or carotid plaque. Coronary artery calcification scoring shows promise in studies that have reported a higher event rate in those with high calcium scores who were assigned to low or intermediate risk by Framingham (38).

Surrogate measures of endothelial function have been used as markers (39–47). These include peripheral arterial tonometry, serum asymmetric dimethylarginine (ADMA), and vascular adhesion molecules (E-selectin). Others are surrogate measures of arterial inflammation, such as highly sensitive C-reactive protein or nitrotyrosine, a specific marker for protein-modification by nitric oxide-derived oxidants, or TNF-alpha. These link inflammation to atherosclerosis development through the nitric oxide pathway. Although the levels of these inflammatory markers are increased in insulin-resistant states of obesity and type 2 diabetes (39, 40), they have not yet been established in the ED literature as predictors of future cardiovascular events. Other markers may include measures of non-HDL-C cholesterol, such as apolipoprotein B (Apo-B), or assessment of "oxidized LDL" cholesterol, part of a group of oxidative damage molecules known as isoprostanes. Lastly, the extremely atherogenic level of small, dense LDL particles (LDL-P) as measured by nuclear magnetic resonance may be of value in risk assessment (48–50). These markers carefully track the functional pathway of impaired endothelial cell dysfunction that is thought to be central to ED and CAD.

Back to Basics: ED and All-Cause Mortality

The Framingham risk score is unique because it is simple, dominated by chronological age, systolic blood pressure, total cholesterol and HDL-C cholesterol, and cigarette smoking. We also know its limitations: the Framingham study involved 5,200 patients from Framingham, Massachusetts, and it is unclear whether this population is applicable to other populations (48). In addition, Framingham does not include triglycerides, family history of cardiac disease, and concepts of exercise and diet, risk factors we know to be of great importance for future cardiovascular disease risk. Therefore I believe that the Framingham risk score underestimates risk and is an inaccurate reflection of true coronary heart disease risk in the ED patient.

One study (51) performed in the Netherlands found that in 1,248 men, free of cardiovascular disease at baseline, 22.8% had reduced erectile rigidity and 8.7% had severely reduced erectile rigidity. During an average of 6.3 years of follow-up, a HR of 1.6 was found for increased cardiovascular events after adjusting for age and cardiovascular disease risk score. In this population-based study, an answer of "yes" to the question about the presence of ED asked at baseline proved to be a predictor of the outcomes of acute myocardial infarction, stroke, and sudden death independent of the Framingham risk factors (51).

A review of 27 studies with 71,727 participants evaluating the accuracy of the Framingham risk score for coronary heart disease found that there was an underprediction of risk in the high-risk population and an overproduction of risk in the lower-risk population (52). This has led to the proposal of other risk scores that factor in additional variables such as family history and lower socioeconomic status (53, 54). However, none of these scoring systems appears clearly superior to the Framingham risk score.

And it is not simply cardiovascular events we are acknowledging. Similar to the Bohm (32) study's findings of increased mortality in ED patients, a recent prospective population-based study of 1,709 men followed for 15 years sought to examine the association of ED with all-cause mortality and cause-specific mortality (55). Mortality due to all causes, including cardiovascular disease, malignant neoplasms, and other causes, was examined. Of these 1,709 men, 1,284 survived to the end of 2004 and had complete ED and age data. Of 403 men who died, 371 had complete data. After adjustment for age, Body Mass Index, alcohol consumption, physical activity, cigarette smoking, self-assessed health and self-reported heart disease, hypertension, and diabetes, ED was associated with HRs of 1.26 (95% CI 1.01–1.57) for all-cause mortality and 1.43 (95% CI 1.00–2.05) for cardiovascular disease mortality. These findings suggest that ED is significantly associated with an increased incidence of all-cause mortality, primarily through its association with cardiovascular disease mortality (55).

Most importantly, the potential use of these novel biomarkers and surrogates, and the acknowledged limitations of the Framingham risk score, begs the question: Can this discovery of increased coronary heart disease risk in the ED patient improve both a man's ED and lessen his overall cardiovascular disease risk? We do not know at present. There remains a lack of correlation between imaging surrogates and outcomes. While biomarkers hold promise for discriminating the vulnerable patient, only a few have been shown to improve prediction independent of conventional risk factors. The ability of high-sensitivity C-reactive protein to identify individuals with higher risk has been noted in the Physicians Health Study and confirmed in other prospective cohorts. One such study promoted an interesting hypothesis to improve risk stratification in Framingham utilizing C-reactive protein and family history (56). Indeed, the Centers for Disease Control and Prevention and the American Heart Association endorsed the use of high-sensitivity C-reactive protein as an adjunct to global risk prediction, particularly in those at "intermediate" risk (57). An elevation in cardiac events in patients with an elevated C-reactive protein level (>2 mg/dL) without LDL elevations was shown in a prospective trial using rosuvastatin (58). Indeed, a recent article by Nozaki and colleagues (59) investigated whether a multiple biomarker strategy that includes plasma levels of endothelium-derived microparticles, reflecting endothelial dysfunction, can improve prediction of future cardiovascular events in high-risk coronary heart disease patients. They used three biomarkers (high-sensitivity C-reactive protein, B-type natriuretic peptide, and endothelium-derived microparticles) in addition to Framingham risk scores in a 36-month prospective study of 387 stable patients at high risk for coronary heart disease and future cardiovascular events. They found that among the 55 patients who developed cardiovascular events, the risk stratification improved when each biomarker or combination of biomarkers was added to the Framingham score (59).

A New Algorithm?

ED is independently correlated with cardiovascular disease risk and is a predictor of future cardiovascular events. Men with ED may obtain a more accurate evaluation of their risk with prudent use of these biomarkers or imaging studies. Only further studies of younger men with ED and preventive measures will provide evidence as to which of the surrogate markers are influential and efficacious in the delineation of this risk.

The typical ED patient has no clinically overt cardiovascular disease. For such patients, investigation for silent CAD and determination of risk for future cardiovascular events is of major importance. Based on popular risk scorings such as the Framingham and Princeton Consensus II (24), a simplified and clinically useful algorithm includes initial stratification of patients to lower (<10% Framingham), higher (>20% Framingham), or intermediate (>10% and <20% Framingham) cardiovascular risk according to the presence or severity of conventional risk factors. We suggest that men without ED and cardiovascular risk factors are at low risk for future cardiovascular events. Men without ED who have cardiovascular risk factors, and men with ED with or without traditional risk factors less than age 60 years thought to be primarily vascular in etiology, should be considered an intermediate-risk group (>10% Framingham) for future cardiovascular events. It is this group of men, especially those under the age of 60 years, who may benefit from the use of some of these surrogate markers of cardiometabolic risk in a cost-effective manner to stratify them for subsequent aggressive treatment of cardiovascular risk factors.

Men at lower risk need lifestyle advice, should have their risk factors addressed, and should be regularly monitored by their primary health care providers (e.g., family doctors Figure 6.2). Those at higher risk, apart from treatment of risk factors, should undergo further cardiologic assessment for reclassification of coronary heart disease risk. Evaluating the pretest likelihood of CAD according to

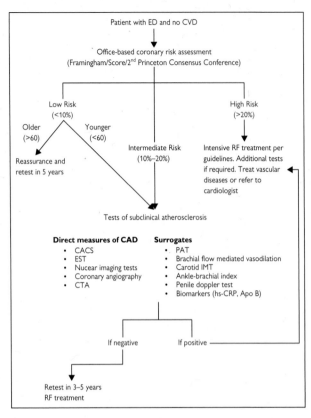

Figure 6.2 Recommended evaluation and management of sardiovascular risk in men with vasculogenic ED but no know cardiovascular disease for the primary care physician. CACS indicates coronary artery calcium score; EST , exercise stress test; CTA, computed tomography with angiogram; PAT, peripheral arterial tonography; IMT, intimal wall thickness; RF, risk factor (60).

the clinical presentation is of utmost importance in the selection of an appropriate diagnostic strategy and interpretation of diagnostic test results. The resting ECG is usually normal, but if it is abnormal, entry into a higher risk category is automatic. As a next step, an exercise ECG is the simplest, most readily available, and least expensive evaluation and is recommended for all men at higher risk. When an exercise ECG is not interpretable (e.g., in the case of a left bundle branch block), when it is inconclusive, or when it cannot be undertaken due to mobility problems, obtaining a scintigraphy perfusion scan or stress echocardiogram is advised. If the stress tests are abnormal, and depending on their exact findings, the option for further evaluation with cardiac angiography emerges.

Ideally, evaluation of patients at intermediate risk should include determination not only of silent CAD but also of risk for developing future CAD events that may be related not only to the development of obstructive lesions, but also to the rupture of vulnerable, nonobstructive plaques. Techniques such as aortic stiffness, carotid ultrasound, ankle–brachial index, flow-mediated dilatation of the brachial artery, peripheral arterial tonometry, penile Doppler flow, coronary calcium scoring, and inflammatory markers/mediators show great potential, and their future implementation is being evaluated according to their individual predictive ability, ease of use, cost, and safety (61). The younger patient (<60 years) with ED may require multiple measures of subclinical atherosclerosis to increase sensitivity for detection of elevated coronary heart disease risk. If these are negative, retesting in 3 to 5 years and aggressive risk-factor reduction should be undertaken.

Conclusion

To answer Thompson's question (4) about whether erectile function could serve as a surrogate measure of the efficacy of preventive interventions for cardiac disease, Inman and Hackett suggest further studies of cardiovascular disease prevention strategies in men with ED. Men with ED may have or may be at risk of developing a potentially serious condition, perhaps a cardiovascular event within 5 to 10 years (4). Therefore, the screening and monitoring of men with ED is not only advisable, but necessary. Only then can we fully comprehend and implement a "window of curability" whereby future cardiac events might be prevented.

Unfortunately, at this time, chronic disease management protocols in primary care in the United States continue to ignore the health importance of ED. Most significant, restricting access to ED treatment in both the United States and Europe by non–evidence-based legislation may prevent many men and their providers from reaping the benefits of early detection and therapy.

Acknowledgments

The author wishes to acknowledge the following individuals upon whose work this manuscript is based: Robert Kloner, MD; Peiro Montorsi, MD; Ajay Nehra, MD, and Graham Jackson, MD.

References

1. Selvin E, Burnett AL, Platz EA. Prevalence and risk factors for erectile dysfunction in the US. *Am J Med* 2007;120:151–157.

2. Miner M, Kuritzky L. Erectile dysfunction: a sentinel marker for cardiovascular disease in primary care. *Cleve Clin J Med* 2007;74:S30–S37.

3. Castelli WP, Abbott RD, McNamara PM. Summary estimates of cholesterol used to predict coronary heart disease. *Circulation* 1983;67(4):730–734.

4. Thompson IM, Tamgen CM, Goodman PJ, Probstfield JL, Moinpour CM, Coltman CA. Erectile dysfunction and subsequent cardiovascular disease. *JAMA* 2005;294:2296–3002.

5. Gazzaruso C, Solerte SB, Pujia A, et al. Erectile dysfunction as a predictor of cardiovascular events and death in diabetic patients with angiographically proven asymptomatic coronary artery disease: a potential protective role for statins and 5-phosphodiesterase inhibitors. *J Am Coll Cardiol* 2008;51(21):2040–2044.

6. Ma RC, So WY, Yang X, et al. Erectile dysfunction predicts coronary artery disease in type 2 diabetics. *J Am Coll Cardiol* 2008;51(21):2045–2050.

7. Inman BA, St. Sauver JL, Jacobson DJ, et al. A population-based longitudinal study of erectile dysfunction and future coronary artery disease. *Mayo Clin Proc.* 2009;84(2):108–113.

8. Miner M. Erectile dysfunction and the "window of curability": A harbinger of cardiovascular events [editorial]. *Mayo Clin Proc* 2009;84(2):102–104.

9. Montorsi P, Montorsi F, Schulman CC. Is erectile dysfunction the "tip of the iceberg" of a systemic vascular disorder? [editorial] *Eur Urol.* 2003;44(3):352–354.

10. Feldman HA, Goldstein I, Hatzichristou D, Krane RJ, McKinlay JB. Impotence and its medical and psychological correlates: results of the Massachusetts Male Aging Study. *J Urol* 1994;151:54–61.

11. Bortolotti A, Parazzini F, Colli E, Landoni M. The epidemiology of erectile dysfunction and its risk factors. *Int J Androl* 1997;20:323–334.

12. Solomon H, Man JW, Wierzbicki AS, Jackson G. Relation of erectile dysfunction to angiographic artery disease. *Am J Cardiol* 2002;91:230–231.

13. Montorsi F, Briganti A, Salonia A, et al. Erectile dysfunction prevalence, time of onset and association with risk factors in 300 consecutive patients with acute chest pain and angiographically documented coronary artery disease. *Eur Urol* 2003;44:360–365.

14. Kloner R, Mullin S, Shook T, et al. Erectile dysfunction in the cardiac patient: how common and should we treat? *J Urol* 2003;170:S46-S50.

15. Montorsi P, Ravagnani PM, Galli S, et al. Association between erectile dysfunction and coronary artery disease. Role of coronary clinical presentation and extent of coronary vessels involvement: the COBRA trial. *Eur Heart J* 2006;27(22):2632–2639.

16. Gazzarusso C, Giordanetti S, De Amici E, et al. Relationship between erectile dysfunction and silent myocardial ischemia in apparently uncomplicated type 2 diabetic patients. *Circulation* 2004;110:22–26.

17. Korpelainenl JT, Kauhanen ML, Kemola H, Malinen U, Myllyla VV. Sexual dysfunction in stoke patients. *Acta Neurol Scand* 1998;98:400–405.

18. Burchard M, Burchard T, Anastasiadis AG, Kiss AJ, Shabsigh A, de La Taille A. Erectile dysfunction is a marker for cardiovascular complications and psychological functioning in men with hypertension. *Int J Impot Res* 2001;13:276–281.

19. Virag R, Bouilly P. Is impotence an arterial disease? A study of arterial risk factors in 440 impotence men. *Lancet* 1985;322:181–184.

20. Azadzoi KM, Goldstein I. Erectile dysfunction due to atherosclerotic vascular disease: the development of an animal model. *J Urol* 1992;147:1675–1681.

21. Azadzoi KM, deTeiada IS. Hypercholesterolemia impairs endothelium-dependent relaxation of rabbit corpus cavernosum smooth muscle. *J Urol* 1991;146:238–240.

22. Solomon H, Man JW, Jackson G. Erectile dysfunction and the cardiovascular patient: endothelial dysfunction is the common denominator. *Heart* 2003;89:179–184.

23. Laumann EO, Palik A, Rosen RC. Sexual dysfunction in the United States: prevalence and predictors. *JAMA* 1999;281:537–544.

24. Jackson G, Rosen RC, Kloner RA, Kostis JB. The second Princeton consensus on sexual dysfunction and cardiac risk: new guidelines for sexual medicine. *J Sex Med.* 2006;3: 28–36.

25. Hackett G. The burden and extent of comorbid conditions in patients with erectile dysfunction. *Int J Clin Pract* 2009;63(8):1205–1213.

26. Kaya C, Uslu Z, Karaman I. Is endothelial function impaired in erectile dysfunction patients? *Int J Impot Res* 2006;18:55–60.

27. Mykletun A, Dahl AA, O'Leary MP, Fossa SD. Assessment of male sexual function by the Brief Sexual Function Inventory. *BJU Int* 2006;97:316–323.

28. Inman BA, Sauver JL, Jacobson DJ, et al. A population-gased longitudinal study of erectile dysfunction and future coronary artery disease. *Mayo Clin Proc* 2009;84(2):108–130.

29. Chew KK, Finn J, GradDip PH, et al. Erectile dysfunction as a predictor for subsequent atherosclerotic cardiovascular events: findings from a linked-data study. *J Sex Med* 2010;7:192–202.

30. O'Rourke MF, Hashimoto J. Mechanical factors in arterial aging: a clinical perspective. *J Am Coll Cardiol.* 2007;50:1–13.

31. Caretta N, Palego P, Ferlin A, et al. Resumption of spontaneous erections in selected patients affected by erectile dysfunction and various degrees of carotid wall alteration: role of tadalafil. *Eur Urol* 2005;48:326–331.

32. Bohm M, Baumhakel M, Teo K, et al for the ONTARGET/TRANSCEND Erectile Dysfunction Substudy Investigators. Erectile dysfunction predicts events in high-risk patients receiving telmisatan, ramipril, or both. *Circulation* 2010;121:1439–1446.

33. Billups KL, Blank AJ, Padma-Nathan H, Katz S, Williams R. Erectile dysfunction is a marker for cardiovascular disease: results of the Minority Health Institute Expert Advisory Panel. *J Sex Med* 2005;2:40–52.

34. Alderman EL, Corley SD, Fisher LD, et al. Five-year angiographic follow-up of factors associated with progression of coronary artery disease in the Coronary Artery Surgery Study (CASS). *J Am Coll Cardiol* 1993;22:1141–1154.

35. Dandona P, Aljada A, Bandyopadhyay A. Inflammation: the link between insulin resistance, obesity and type 2 diabetes. *Trends Immunol* 2004;25:4–7.

36. Barter P, Gotto AM, LaRosa JC, Maroni J, et al. HDL cholesterol, very low levels of LDL cholesterol, and cardiovascular events. *N Engl J Med* 2007;357(13):1301–1310.

37. Giugliano F, Esposito K, Di Palo C, et al. Erectile dysfunction associates with endothelial dysfunction and raised proinflammatory cytokine levels in obese men. *J Endocrin Invest* 2004;27:665–669.

38. Detrano R, Guerci AD, Carr JJ, et al. Coronary calcium as a predictor of coronary events in four racial or ethnic groups. *N Engl J Med* 2008;358:1336–1345.

39. Dandona P, Aljada A, Bandyopadhyay A. Inflammation: the link between insulin resistance, obesity and type 2 diabetes. *Trends Immunol* 2004;25:4–7.

40. Esposito K, Giugliano F, Martedi E, et al. High proportions of erectile dysfunction in men with the metabolic syndrome. *Diabetes Care* 2005;28:1201–1203.

41. Vlachopoulos C, Konstantinos R, Ioakeimidis N, et al. Inflammation, metabolic syndrome, erectile dysfunction and coronary artery disease: common links. *Eur Urol* 2007;52:1590–1600.

42. Billups KL, Kaiser DR, Kelly AS, et al. Relation of C-reactive protein and other cardiovascular risk factors to penile vascular disease in men with erectile dysfunction. *Int J Impot Res* 2003;15:231–236.

43. Bocchio M, Desideri G, Scarpelli P, et al. Endothelial cell activation in men with erectile dysfunction without cardiovascular risk factors and overt vascular damage. *J Urol* 2004;171:1601–1604.

44. Sullivan ME, Miller MA, Bell CR, et al. Fibrinogen, lipoprotein (a) and lipids in patients with erectile dysfunction. *Int Angiol* 2001;20:195–199.

45. Giugliano F, Esposito K, Di Palo C, et al. Erectile dysfunction associates with endothelial dysfunction and raised proinflammatory cytokine levels in obese men. *J Endocrin Invest* 2004;27:665–669.

46. Eaton CB, Liu YL, Mittleman MA, et al. A retrospective study of the new relationship between biomarkers of atherosclerosis and erectile dysfunction in 988 men. *Int J Impot Res* 2007;19:218–225.

47. Vlachopoulos C, Aznaouridis K, Ioakeimidis N, et al. Unfavourable endothelial and inflammatory state in erectile dysfunction patients with or without coronary artery disease. *Eur Heart J* 2006;27:2640–2648.

48. D'Agostino RB, Grundy S, Sullivan LM, Wilson P. Validation of the Framingham Heart Disease Prediction Score: results of a multiple ethnic groups investigation. *JAMA* 2001;286:180–187.

49. Cromwell WC, Otvos JD. Low-density lipoprotein particle number and risk for cardiovascular disease. *Curr Athero Rep* 2004;6:381–387.

50. Davidson MH. Editorial: Is LDL-C past its prime? The emerging role of non-HDL, LDL-P, and ApoB in CHD risk assessment. *Arterioscler Thromb Vasc Biol* 2008;28:1582–1583.

51. Schouten BWV, Bohnen AM, Bosch JL, et al. Erectile dysfunction prospectively associated with cardiovascular disease in the Dutch general population: results from the Krimpen Study. *Int J Impot Res* 2008;20(1):9.

52. Brindle P, Beswick A, Fahey T, Ebrahim S. Accuracy and impact of risk assessment in the primary prevention of cardiovascular disease: a systemic review. *Heart* 2006;92:1752–1759.

53. Hippisley-Cox J, Coupland C, Vinogradova Y, et al. Derivation and validation of QRISK, a new cardiovascular risk score for the United Kingdom: prospective open cohort study. *BMJ* 2007;335:136–148.

54. Woodward M, Brindle P, Tunstall-Pedoe H. Adding social deprivation and family history to the cardiovascular risk assessment: the ASSIGN score form the Scottish Heart Health Extended Cohort (SHHEC). *Heart* 2007;2:172–176.

55. Araujo AB, Travison TG, Ganz PA, et al. Erectile dysfunction and mortality. *J Sex Med* 2009 [E-pub before print].

56. Ridker PM. C-reactive protein and the prediction of cardiovascular events among those at intermediate risk: moving an inflammatory hypothesis toward consensus. *J Am Coll Cardiol* 2007;49:2129–2138.

57. Pearson TA, Mensah GA, Alexander RW, et al. Markers of inflammation and cardiovascular disease: application to clinical and public health practice: a statement for healthcare professionals from the Centers for Disease Control and Prevention and the American Heart Association. *Circulation* 2003;107:499–511.

58. Ridker PM, Danielson E, Fonseca FAH, et al. for the JUPITER Study Group. Rosuvastatin to prevent vascular events in men and women with elevated C-reactive protein. *N Engl J Med* 2008;359:2195–2207.

59. Nozaki T, Sugiyama S, Hidenobu K, et al. Significance of multiple biomarkers strategy including endothelial dysfunction to improve risk stratification for cardiovascular events in patients at high risk for coronary heart disease. *J Am Coll Cardiol* 2009;54:601–608.

60. Miner M. Erectile Dysfunction: A Harbinger or Consequence: Does Its Detection Lead to a Window of Curability? *J Androl* 2010;32(2).

61. Montorsi P, Ravagnani P, Galli S, et al. Association between erectile dysfunction and coronary artery disease: matching the right target with the right test in the right patient. *Eur Urol* 2006;50:721–731.

Chapter 7

A Multidisciplinary Approach to Erectile Dysfunction

Dioma U. Udeoji, Waguih William IsHak, Konstantin Balayan, Ashraf Ismail, and Ernst R. Schwarz

Erectile dysfunction (ED) is a highly prevalent condition, affecting more than 50% of men over the age of 60 (1), and it is projected to affect more than 300 million men worldwide by 2025 (2). Sexual function involves anatomy, physiology, endocrinology, individual behavior, and couples' dynamics, as well as sociocultural influences (3). ED is a multifactorial problem of vasculogenic, pharmacological, neurological, hormonal, surgical, medical, and psychological origin. These factors are outlined below and require a goal-driven, multidisciplinary management approach.

Vasculogenic Causes

Most ED cases are vasculogenic in nature (4). In patients with underlying cardiovascular disorders, vascular causes play an even larger role in the development of ED. Vasculogenic causes of ED can be subdivided into venous insufficiency, arterial insufficiency, and endothelial dysfunction. Atherosclerosis appears to be present in 40% of ED cases in men more than 50 years of age (5) and might contribute to reduced arterial inflow into the penile corpora cavernosa (6). Smoking appears to be a significant risk factor for ED because of its atherogenic effects causing vascular insufficiency and a decrease in penile nitric oxide (NO) levels (2, 7). Other modifiable risk factors for ED are diabetes mellitus, hypertension, hyperlipidemia, obesity, and sedentary lifestyle.

Endothelial dysfunction appears to be a systemic phenomenon, affecting both the coronary and peripheral circulation. Oxygen-derived free radicals have also been associated with inhibition of endothelium-dependent vasodilation, suggesting that rapid inactivation of NO may be caused by increased free radical production (8). Other possible mechanisms of endothelial dysfunction include cell surface receptor abnormalities or alterations at the G protein level, which may account for decreased efficacy of free NO, as seen in atherosclerosis (9).

Pharmacological Causes

ED can be caused by medications and drugs (2, 10). Beta-adrenergic receptor blockers, commonly used for the treatment of hypertension, coronary artery disease, and heart failure, are known to have negative effects on male sexual function (11). Theories point to the adverse effects of decreased perfusion pressure or a direct (but unknown) effect on smooth muscle. Support for the latter mechanism is derived from the observation that despite pressure-lowering effects, treatment with alpha-adrenergic receptor blockers is not associated with ED, and that this class of medications may actually improve ED (12).

Atenolol (13), propranolol (14), and metoprolol (15) have been associated with ED, but some reports reveal negative effects with most if not all beta-adrenergic beta-receptor blockers. It is also believed that beta-blockers can cause (or worsen) depression, and depression itself might also play a role in the occurrence of ED; however, there is controversy and clinical trials do not support this hypothesis (16).

While ED caused by diuretics has been reported, the mechanism remains poorly defined (11). More than 10% of patients taking thiazide diuretics may experience a decline in sexual function (17).

The impact of angiotensin-converting enzyme (ACE) inhibitors and angiotensin II receptor blockers on ED is unclear. Croog and colleagues found that the ACE inhibitor captopril actually enhances sexual function (14). Interestingly, if ACE inhibitor therapy (e.g., for the treatment of heart failure) is associated with an improved functional cardiac status, this might result in improved sexual function (18), at least in a subset of patients.

Other common medications associated with ED are:

1. Antidepressants
   A. Tricyclics, such as desipramine, maprotiline, nortriptyline (inhibit ejaculation), amitriptyline, protriptyline, doxepin, imipramine (inhibit ejaculation and also cause impotence), amoxapine (decreases libido and also causes impotence)
   B. Monoamine oxidase (MAO) inhibitors, such as isocarboxazid, tranylcypromine (inhibit ejaculation), phenelzine (inhibits ejaculation and deceases libido), atypical agent such as trazodone (causes priapism)
2. Antipsychotics
   A. Selective serotonin reuptake inhibitors (SSRIs), such as perphenazine, trifluoperazine (inhibit ejaculation), fluoxetine (causes anorgasmia in 8% of patients)
   B. Phenothiazines, such as fluphenazine, mesoridazine (inhibit ejaculation and decrease libido), chlorpromazine (inhibits ejaculation), thioridazine (inhibits ejaculation, decreases libido, and causes priapism)
   C. Thioxanthene, such as chlorprothixene (inhibits ejaculation), thiothixene (inhibits ejaculation and can cause impotence)
   D. Lithium (can cause impotence)
   E. Haloperidol (inhibits ejaculation)
3. Antifungal, such as ketoconazole (causes impotence)
4. Antiulcer medications, such as cimetidine (can decrease libido, can cause impotence and gynecomastia)
5. Cholesterol-lowering agents
6. Hormonal drugs, such as finasteride and dutasteride

7. Cocaine
8. Heroin
9. Alcohol
10. Marijuana (2)

The above side effects are not very common but can occur in some patients.

Neurological Causes

Most neurological problems, such as cerebrovascular accident, multiple sclerosis (2, 19, 20), Guillain-Barré syndrome, seizure disorders, Alzheimer's disease, Parkinson's disease, and brain and spinal cord injuries, can lead to ED because of damage to the nerves that transmit impulses from the brain to the spinal cord and then to the penis. Pelvic injuries or diseases can damage the nerves, vessels, or both needed for penile erection, thereby causing ED (2).

Endocrine and Hormonal Causes

Hormonal imbalances can lead to ED. The pathogenesis is multifactorial and can be secondary to kidney or liver pathology (2, 7). A progressive decline in the serum testosterone level occurs with normal aging. Studies have demonstrated that men with moderate to severe hypogonadism suffer from at least one form of sexual disorder, such as decreased libido, impaired seminal emission, ejaculatory problems, ED, and decreased frequency and a reduction in the magnitude of nocturnal erection. Longitudinal data from the Massachusetts Male Aging Study demonstrated that the prevalence of symptomatic hypogonadism in men between the ages of 40 and 69 years is between 6% and 12% (21–23). The prevalence of endocrine problems as a cause of sexual disorder has risen from 2% to 23% (24). Most hormonal causes of ED revolve around the hypothalamic-pituitary-gonadal axis. Interruption of this axis can lead to endocrine disorders such as hyperprolactinemia or hypogonadism (2). Medication use can also result to hyperprolactinemia, which may eventually result in ED. Other endocrine causes, such as thyroid diseases, adrenal insufficiency, acromegaly, diabetes mellitus, Cushing's syndrome, congenital problems (e.g., myotonic dystrophy, Klinefelter's syndrome, Kallmann's syndrome), unilateral mumps orchitis (which results in failure of normal function of the testis later in life), and autoimmune destruction of the testis (2), can result in ED or other forms of sexual disorder.

Medical Causes

Many medical diseases can predispose men to ED. The most common chronic disease conditions are diabetes mellitus and hypertension, probably due to the neurovascular and microvascular changes associated with these conditions (2). Urological causes (e.g., benign prostatic hyperplasia, Peyronie's disease) as well as many other chronic organic dysfunctions or diseases, such as chronic renal failure, heart failure, liver failure, sickle cell anemia, coronary artery disease, leukemias, cancers, chronic obstructive pulmonary diseases, zinc deficiency, malnutrition (2, 25), chronic fatigue, frailty, and old age, can lead to ED.

Surgical Causes

Surgical procedures or irradiation affecting the pelvic organs (such as the prostate, bladder, rectum, and colon) and retroperitoneal organs can lead to ED due to damage to the blood vessels and nerves responsible for erection. Also, trauma or surgical procedures on the brain and spinal cord can lead to ED due to damage to the nerves and neurons that relay impulses from the brain to the spinal cord and then to the penis (2).

Psychosocial Causes

Psychological problems such as depression, anxiety, stress, fatigue, sadness, guilt (especially about sex), and bereavement can all lead to any kind of sexual disorder. Psychological causes of ED are of rapid onset, and ED can resolve as soon as the psychological problem is resolved. The presence of early morning erection suggests a psychological cause of ED rather than an organic cause (2).

The Multidisciplinary Team Approach

The existence of more than one of these causes of ED requires more than a simplified organic approach to manage ED. A multidisciplinary team approach involves bringing together multiple disciplines to redefine multifaceted cases (such as ED) and reach solutions based on a new understanding of complex medical conditions. In the 1960s, Bonita (an anesthesiologist) founded the first multidisciplinary clinic involving neurologists, internists, neurosurgeons, orthopaedic surgeons, and psychologists for the management of patients with chronic pain. He was prompted to form a multidisciplinary clinic due to his frustration in treating patients with chronic/persistent pain. Over the years many hospitals adopted his approach, and some institutions and professional societies produced guidelines centered on a multidisciplinary approach to managing multifaceted health issues such as ED, obesity, prostate cancer, fibromyalgia, diabetes mellitus, and multiple sclerosis (4, 19, 26, 27). The members of the multidisciplinary team provide a comprehensive assessment through their individual expertise and in consultation with one another. The approach promotes coordination and communication and can save the patient the stress of undergoing separate and multiple evaluations, multiple interpretations, and multiple treatment plans. In the multidisciplinary approach, differences of opinion can be discussed and resolved as a team. This usually offers the patient the highest standard of care and deters him from interpreting and deciding upon differing viewpoints.

The benefits of a multidisciplinary team approach to patient care are enormous. It gives the patient the confidence that the health professionals are all communicating and working together in regard to his health condition. This approach takes the burden off the patient (i.e., the burden of sharing information that he may not fully understand) and places it instead on the health care professionals, who are better able to deal with the information and use it correctly to manage the patient. In the multidisciplinary approach, the patient is usually at the center of the management, while the health care professionals and family members (if he chooses to involve them) surround him to provide care and support.

A multidisciplinary approach benefits not only the patient but also the health care team. They have the opportunity to enhance their professional skills and knowledge by learning more about the disease and the strategies used by various specialties. A multidisciplinary team approach includes a built-in consultation component that provides medical professionals with ongoing support, which can be invaluable as they deal with many multifaceted cases. The team members work together to develop a treatment plan and strategy and then combine their efforts to provide the highest standard of care for the patient.

A multidisciplinary team approach to the management of ED might involve a cardiologist, a neurologist, a urologist, an endocrinologist, a psychiatrist, a vascular surgeon, a sex therapist, and a psychologist (3, 10, 28). In 1987, Gall and colleagues proposed a multidisciplinary approach to ED (4). A multidisciplinary investigation was performed on 136 patients with ED. The study demonstrated that 85% of the ED cases were organic; 76% were due to vascular causes (4). An international consultant, together with major urological and medical societies, gathered more than 200 multidisciplinary specialists from 60 countries, and they developed guidelines for the management of ED that focused on a multidisciplinary team approach (29). Other professional societies, such as the International Consultation of Sexual Medicine (ICSM-5) have developed an evidence-based multidisciplinary team approach to sexual disorders, including ED; disorders of orgasm, libido, and ejaculation; priapism; and Peyronie's disease (28). In 2005 Schwarz and colleagues developed a multidisciplinary approach to assess ED in high-risk cardiovascular patients (10). In this approach, a cardiologist, a urologist, a psychiatrist, and a vascular surgeon came together to develop an initial assessment program for these patients. The authors proposed a 10-step program called the "Sex and the Heart" evaluation (Table 7.1). Each of the 10 steps is scored, and then the scores are summed to produce a total (risk) score.

The 10 steps involve the following:

1. To increase awareness about potential sexual problems in patients with cardiovascular disorders, to try to make patients comfortable talking about their sexual problems, and to describe their concerns
2. Evaluation of potential causes such as cardiovascular risk factors, illicit drugs (e.g., cocaine), diabetes, smoking history, and drug side effects, as well as ruling out primarily urological causes (e.g., Peyronie's disease), psychiatric causes (e.g., anxiety, depression, or side effects of antidepressants, antipsychotic medications, or mood stabilizers), medical causes (e.g., multiple sclerosis, fibromyalgia, history of cerebrovascular accident,

Table 7.1		Management for Men at Risk for ED: Sex and the Heart
STEP 1	1	**S**exual performance description (discussion)
	2	**E**valuation of potential causes (medication use)
	3	E**X**ercise capacity (stress test)
	4	**a**ssessment of contributing factors
	5	**t**eam approach (PUPSTC)
STEP 2	6	Control concomitant **H**ealth conditions
	7	Optimize **E**F
	8	**A**ugment perfusion (vasculogenic ED)
	9	Reduce **R**isk factors
	10	Follow-up + alternative **T**herapy

With permission, Ernst R Schwarz, *Sex and the Heart, What women need to know about erectile dysfunction*, Friedel & Ernst Academic Press, Los Angeles, California & Haldorf, Germany, ISBN 0–9786846–0–5, 2006

sickle cell anemia, blood dyscrasias such as leukemia), or surgical causes (e.g., pelvic injuries, irradiation, or surgeries)

3. Evaluation of cardiac capacity: functional status assessment, eventually baseline ECG, echocardiography, baseline brain natriuretic peptide (BNP) and exercise stress testing, if clinically indicated

4. Assessment of contributing factors, such as risk factors or others that are not considered to be the primary cause of ED but potentially worsen sexual function (e.g., chronically elevated blood sugar levels in a diabetic patient who also smokes). Other diagnostic tests, when indicated, can be performed to evaluate the factors contributing to ED: sensory studies (biothesiometry), nocturnal penile tumescence and rigidity test (Snap-Gauge test, nocturnal penile tumescence monitoring using the RigiScan), bloodwork (serum testosterone and prolactin level, blood chemistry to rule out anemia, kidney diseases, and thyroid diseases), vascular assessment (penile color duplex ultrasonography, Penile Brachial Index, pharmaco-cavernosometry, cavernosography) (2, 26)

5. Combined evaluation by the entire team involved in the patient's care (ideally, primary care physician, urologist, psychiatrist or psychologist, sexual therapist, and cardiologist or vascular specialist [PUPSTC])

6. Control of concomitant health conditions (e.g., blood pressure control, tight glycemic control, adequate treatment of hyperlipidemia, weight reduction in overweight and obese patients)

7. Attempt to stabilize clinical condition and to improve cardiac capacity (in patients with underlying heart failure), which is usually carried out by adherence to American Heart Association/American College of Cardiology guidelines (e.g., for the management of heart failure), since improved cardiac function can result in improved physical and sexual activity levels

8. Augmentation of regional perfusion, in particular in cases with proven vascular components. This can be performed by assessment of the vascular anatomy and/or regional perfusion studies and, in rare cases, followed by interventional or surgical procedures such as percutaneous transluminal

angioplasty of the iliac arteries or direct penile revascularization surgery or—more frequently—by use of phosphodiesterase-5 (PDE-5) inhibitors (if there are no contraindications such as concomitant use of nitrates)

9. Active reduction of (vascular) risk factors (e.g., smoking cessation, cessation of illicit drug use), with particular emphasis on sexual function. Interestingly, more patients quit smoking for fear of its negative effects on sexual function than its effects on cardiac function.

10. Regular follow-up visits are required in most cases, in particular because more than one treatment attempt or dose adjustments in PDE-5 inhibitor therapy might be required in individual patients. In unsuccessful cases, alternative treatment options should be considered. In contrast to the multidisciplinary approach for the initial assessment, follow-up is scheduled by one practitioner, either the patient's primary care physician or the cardiologist or urologist, depending on the primary problem or primary treatment plan.

Zamboni argued that it is vital to involve a sex therapist (as part of the multidisciplinary team approach) to assess and treat the nonmedical causes of ED (30).

Treatment Options

Oral PDE-5 Inhibitors

In March 1998, sildenafil citrate (Viagra) became the first oral drug for ED approved in the United States. Sildenafil and other PDE-5 inhibitors enhance cGMP-NO-mediated vasodilatation. Detumescence occurs when type 5 phosphodiesterase catabolizes cGMP, accompanied by NO depletion and restoration of penile vascular tone. PDE-5 inhibitors thereby increase both the number and duration of erections in men. In a quantitative meta-analysis of 27 trials in 6,659 men with ED, a higher percentage of successful sexual intercourse was achieved with sildenafil compared with placebo (57% vs. 21%, respectively) (31).

Patient education is critical for an optimal response to sildenafil. This includes informing the patient to take the medication on an empty stomach and to time sexual activity so that it occurs within 1 to 6 hours after intake. Peak serum concentration occurs at 1 hour, and drug half-life is 4 to 5 hours.

Vardenafil (Levitra) and tadalafil (Cialis) are newer phosphodiesterase inhibitors that appear to be as effective as sildenafil (32, 33). Tadalafil has a longer duration of action, offering the hypothetical advantage of allowing more spontaneity in sexual activity. Like sildenafil, they both also potentiate the hypotensive response to nitrates. Therefore, all PDE-5 inhibitors are contraindicated in patients taking concomitant nitrate or any NO donor (nitroprusside, nitroglycerine, molsidomine) caution is advised for some PDE-5 inhibitors and concomittant alpha blocker use even though it is not contra-indicated (34,35).

Common side effects include headache, flushing, nasal congestion, allergic reactions, indigestion, migraine, rhinorrhea, back pain, and myalgias. Most of these side effects are transient.

Other Oral Drugs

Other oral drugs for treatment of ED are apomorphine (Apokyn) and yohimbine (Yocon). Apomorphine is centrally acting and has shown mild clinical efficacy in the treatment of ED (36). Currently it is not available in the United States, but it is available in several European and Middle Eastern countries. Yohimbine is an alpha-2 receptor blocker with limited efficacy in the treatment of ED (37). It should be used with caution because of its cardiovascular side effects, including tachycardia and the potential for hypertension. Despite aggressive marketing, there are no data to support the assertion that nutritional supplements, herbal therapy, or vitamins have a beneficial effect in the treatment of ED (38).

Oral phentolamine (Vasomax) is an alpha-adrenergic blocking agent used to treat mild to moderate ED. It is not as effective as PDE-5 inhibitors, but it has a faster onset of action and little or no interaction with nitrates. Side effects are hypotension, headache, nausea, lightheadedness, and nausea (35).

Opioid antagonists such as naltrexone may be helpful in treating ED in patients with poor libido (35). They are contraindicated in patients who have used any narcotics within the past 10 days. High doses of naltrexone can cause liver damage.

A study demonstrated that 88% of hypertensive men with sexual disorders reported improvement in at least one sexual function domain after 12 weeks of therapy with an angiotensin-receptor blocker, such as losartan. A Japanese study reported that patients less than 65 years old had improved sexual function when they switched to candesartan (39).

Trazodone (serotonin receptor reuptake inhibitor) improves premature ejaculation and erectile function in men with psychogenic ED (35, 40).

Isoxsuprine is a vasodilator that acts by stimulating beta-adrenergic receptors, thereby causing relaxation of vascular smooth muscle (35, 41).

A relative old concept based on the pathophysiology has recently been rediscovered, which is the supplementation of nitric oxide as a direct (penile) vasodilator. Nitric oxide, a gas, has recently been approved and made available as a supplement (NEO40[(TM)]) in the from of a lozenge, which delivers the nitric oxide gas in the mouth. Usage has been anecdotally reported to improve penile perfusion, improve erections and booster the effects of PDE-5 inhibitors, but should be taken one hour after or befoe the consumption of PDE-5 inhibitors. Our initial experience has been extraordinary, but further large scale studies are required to verify these promising results.

Hormonal Therapy

Treatment of hypogonadism results in feelings of enhanced sexuality and reliable improvement in the symptoms of decreased libido. Male hypogonadism can be treated with testosterone replacement therapy in form of a gel, patch, pellet, or oral or injectable testosterone esters. Testosterone replacement therapy in men with secondary hypogonadism results in improvements in sexual function, motivation, desire, mood, performance, muscle strength, lean body mass, fat distribution, and body composition (42). However, pure vasculogenic or neurogenic ED may not respond well to replacement therapy if hormonal insufficiency is not the main cause of ED.

Invasive Treatment Modalities

Penile injections with vasoactive medications are effective in 70% to 80% of patients; they have an onset of action within 10 minutes and are relatively painless

(43). They are used by approximately 10% of patients with ED and are the most common treatment for men who take nitrates or those who have had no success with PDE-5 inhibitors. Alprostadil (prostaglandin E1) is the most frequently used. The overall risk is relatively low: there has only been one case report of myocardial infarction temporally associated with alprostadil penile injection. There is no cardiovascular contraindication to its use, but there is an increased injection-induced bleeding risk in patients who are on chronic anticoagulation (44). Other common agents used are a combination of alprostadil, phentolamine, and papaverine (Trimix) (19, 35). These agents have been studied in patients with traumatic spinal cord injury, and they are equally effective in other forms of ED, especially neurogenic ED. Some studies reported a 95% success rate in patients with ED secondary to traumatic spinal cord injury (45). The success rate is defined as a penile erection adequate for achieving vaginal penetration. Of interest, most patients with traumatic spinal cord injury are highly sensitive to vasodilators and therefore should use a low dose of vasodilators (19).

Thymoxamine (Moxisylyte) is a selective alpha-1-adrenergic receptor antagonist used in the treatment of ED. This agent is very effective and has a low side-effect profile (35).

Vasoactive polypeptide and phentolamine (Invicorp) is used in the treatment of ED in countries such as Denmark but is not approved for use in the United States. The most common side effects are tachycardia and flushing (35).

Intraurethral suppositories of alprostadil avoid penile injection but are less effective and have increased adverse effects (19, 45). The most common adverse effect is penile pain (12%); other side effects are dizziness, testicular pain, and urethral bleeding. This technique requires placing a tourniquet at the base of the penis for optimal results (46). Initial treatment should take place in a health care or monitored environment owing to the rare occurrence of syncope.

Intercavernosal injection therapy produces erections in more than 85% of the patients, but compliance is low, with a dropout rate of up to 50%.

Mechanical Devices

Vacuum constriction devices offer a noninvasive mechanical alternative and are used worldwide by approximately 5% of men with ED (47). A plastic cylinder is placed around the penis that draws blood into the penis by creating negative pressure. A tourniquet is placed at the base of the penis once adequate rigidity is attained, trapping blood within the corpora cavernosa. When vacuum erection devices were used in patients with spinal cord injury, 93% and 76% of the patients achieved an erection adequate for vaginal penetration at 3 months and 6 months of therapy, respectively (48). Common adverse effects in the spinal cord injury population were premature loss of erection, abrasions, discomfort, petechiae, ecchymosis, leg spasms, and skin edema (19, 48).

Electrical stimulation devices such as transanal pelvic plexus stimulation and percutaneous perineal electrostimulation are promising noninvasive treatment options under investigation for the treatment of ED. Vibratory stimulation, electrostimulation of the glans penis, or rectal probe electrostimulation can induce erection and ejaculation in patients with neurogenic ED (19). Additional agents can sometimes be used to augment their effects.

Adjunct Therapies

Some adjunct therapies that seem to be helpful in the management of sexual dysfunction are sex therapy, psychosexual counseling, family support, lifestyle modification, risk factor modification, and gene therapy.

Surgical Implants

Surgical implants remain a successful and satisfying treatment for men whose condition has failed to respond to oral therapy and who find other treatment options unsatisfactory (49). Nevertheless, the number of procedures performed is relatively low compared with the estimated population with ED. The primary risks are mechanical device failure (2% at 2 years, 14% at 5 years) and infection (2–3% of cases) (49, 50). In particular, in patients with a cardiac history or known vascular disorders and concomitant associated higher operative risks, most urologists do not recommend device implantation. This also represents the last-resort ED treatment, since it excludes all other treatment options and therefore should be reserved for a highly selected group of patients who failed to respond to all other treatment options, after minimizing all surgical risks.

Psychiatry and Psychology

The role of psychiatry, psychology, and psychiatric social work in sexual medicine is vital to the success of the treatment team approach in erectile dysfunction (ED). In the DSM-IV TR (51), male erectile disorder is defined as inability to attain or to maintain an adequate erection until the completion of the sexual activity. The overall prevalence of ED ranges from 10-52% (52). Biological and psychosocial factors and/or their combination are responsible for ED. Psychosocial factors are very important to detect and treat. ED is not uncommon in individuals with psychiatric disorders such Mood Disorders especially depression, Anxiety Disorders, and Psychotic Disorders. Performance anxiety is known to interfere with ability to obtain and maintain erection. ED is associated with patients who experienced significant stressors such as traumas, losses, and conflicts in addition to financial, vocational, and residential factors. Relational issues such as lack of attractiveness to the partner, relationship conflicts, and lack of adequacy of sexual stimulation are important causes of ED. Impairment in knowledge, deficient skills, and poor attitude could negatively affect sexual functioning. Knowledge about the anatomy, and physiology of sexual organs cannot be overemphasized. Sexual skills need to be addressed during treatment. Attitude towards sex might be impaired by upbringing, fear of pregnancy, and doubts about the future of the relationship. Another important issue to evaluate with the couple is their commitment and motivation to ameliorate the sexual problem. Individuals who are engaged in extra-relational sexual activities or those who are no longer interested in their partner should not be enrolled in sex therapy. The evaluation is not complete without a full diagnostic work-up that may include laboratory tests, imaging studies, and various interdisciplinary consultations.

Psychosocial interventions are considered a first line treatment for psychological or combined ED and they could be used in combination with medical or surgical treatments. Starting with communication and education, discussing erection and its physiology helps men and their partners understand the problem and provide reassurance about treatment interventions and prognosis. Education often provides immediate relief and helps prepare the couple for the treatment course. The primary psychosocial intervention is Sex Therapy or Sensate Focus Exercises originally developed by Masters and Johnson to assist couples experiencing sexual problems as fully detailed below. Despite being originally introduced by Masters and Johnson as a highly effective therapeutic modality for single men, sex surrogate therapy (53) is no longer recommended by the majority of practicing sex therapists due to the unresolved controversy surrounding its use. Other psychosocial interventions include couple therapy, and individual therapy. Couple therapy helps develop more insights into the dynamics of their relationship and enhance communication. Behavioral techniques such as 'active listening', 'talking and listening exercises', 'assertiveness training', 'role playing', are usually utilized (54). Individual psychotherapy (Supportive, Psychodynamic, Cognitive-Behavioral, Behavioral, or Interpersonal) helps define more clearly the issues within the individual and enhance coping skills (55). Group psychotherapy is for patients with psychiatric disorders, co-morbid medical conditions, substance abuse, and those coping with life stressors or trauma. Financial, vocational and social work consultations are needed to address significant concerns of the patients such as money, living situations and career problems.

Sex Therapy

Originally developed by Masters and Johnson Sex therapy is a psychosocial therapy that focuses on the sexual relationship of the couple involving increased awareness of pleasurable body sensations exercises named collectively Sensate focus. Sensate focus is a series of specific exercises for couples, which encourages each partner to take turns paying increased attention to their own senses.

In the first stage, the couple takes turns touching each other's body, excluding the breasts and genitals. The purpose of the touching is not necessary sexual but to heighten awareness of sensations while touching or being touched by the partner. There is no particular order or expectations of what would please the partner. This the process by which each of the partners will learn more in depth about these issues when they process the exercises in their next therapist appointment. The couple is prohibited from having intercourse, if sexual arousal does occur; they are instructed to masturbate individually afterwards if the urge cannot be resisted. Masters and Johnson recommended silence so that couple could focus on physical sensations.

Sensate focus II is the following stage where the breasts and genitals are now included (and not focused on or started with) in the pleasurable touching routines. The couple learns through meeting with their therapist about their heightened physical sensation awareness, their 'hot spots' and they will learn new techniques such as 'hand guiding'. By having one hand on top of the partner's hand while being touched, the partner could communicate non-verbally regarding more or less pressure, a faster or slower pace, or a change to a different spot.

In the next phase of sensate focus, mutual touching is introduced, and as the couple progresses genito-genital touch is added using the female-on-top position without attempting insertion of the penis into the vagina. For heterosexual couples, the penis (regardless the state of erection) is rubbed against the vulva, clitoris, and vaginal opening. As the couple is more comfortable with more intense contacts without rushing into sexual intercourse (which remains prohibited), insertion of a semi-erected penis could be tried with moving to non-genital touching if arousal becomes too intense and orgasm is impending. More sessions of this level would be processed with the therapist and then the couple is allowed to have full intercourse.

Team Approach

One important paradigm in integrating the interdisciplinary team approach is the application of the Biopsychosocial Model (56). Using principles of general system theory, an American psychiatrist George Engel developed the biopsychosocial model where mental disorders occur within individuals who are part of the whole system. According to Engel, this system has sub-personal (nervous system, cell, molecules) and supra-personal (relationship, community, society) elements. Sexual behavior almost always involves a partner (a real or imaginary). Thus, attempts to evaluate and treat sexual dysfunction using only sub-personal elements (biological or biomedical) will not address the issue completely. Biopsychosocial approach will evaluate sexual disorders by engaging both partners and examining both the cause and its effect on the relationship. Applying the Biopsychosocial Model involves identifying and addressing predisposing, precipitating, and perpetuating factors of erectile dysfunction on the biological (e.g., hormonal), and psychosocial (e.g., depression) dimensions. It would also entail engaging not only individuals but also both partners and, examining and addressing their relationship with its emotional and physical aspects.

Biological factors of erectile dysfunction (ED) would need to be investigated and addressed. These factors include age, genetic predisposition, effects of substances (such as alcohol, illicit drugs, prescription and over the counter medications, dietary supplements and herbs in addition to toxins), and medical conditions both generalized or localized (such as congenital anomalies, neuropathic and vasculopathic problems, endocrinal and hormonal imbalances). For further evaluation and treatment three very important diagnoses will need to be ruled out or detected:

A. An axis I Psychiatric Disorder that better accounts for the sexual disorder
B. A Substance-Induced Sexual Dysfunction
C. A Sexual Dysfunction Due to a General Medical Condition

As the biopsychosocial treatment plan is initiated, biological interventions would include the treatment of psychiatric disorders, medical conditions, identifying and/or replacing agents responsible for ED, and ultimately administer oral medications (such as Phosphodiestrase-5 inhibitors, non PDE-5 agents, hormones), injections, pellets, implants, or devices. Team members responsible for evaluating and addressing the above factors include primary care physicians, Urologists, cardiologists, endocrinologists, and surgeons.

In the presence or absence of biological factors, psychosocial factors would need to bedetected and treated as well. Psychiatrists are responsible for the treatment of psychiatric disordersand side effects of psychiatric medications.

Psychologists participate in the team by providing education, sex therapy, couple therapy, and individual psychotherapy.

Conclusion

ED is a multifactorial problem with several contributing factors, such as vasculogenic, neurogenic, urological, hormonal, medical, psychological, surgical, and pharmacological causes. More than 70% of ED cases are vascular in nature (4). A multidisciplinary approach that is broader than formerly recommended (57) (the previous recommendation called for only a cardiologist, urologist, and psychiatrist) is now recommended to evaluate high-risk patients with ED. This broader approach involving specialists such a vascular surgeon, a cardiologist, a urologist, an endocrinologist, a neurologist, a psychologist/psychiatrist, and a sex therapist as part of the team seems to be more beneficial in the treatment of ED. Treatment options include addressing the vasculogenic causes (by improving cardiac function and regional perfusion and lowering cardiovascular risks); replacing medications with unfavorable side effects on sexual function; treating concomitant medical, neurological, urological, hormonal, surgical, and psychological conditions; modifying lifestyle/risk factors; and trying PDE-5 inhibitors. Involving the patient's family to provide support seems to be beneficial in the management of ED.

References

1. Jackson G, Rosen RC, Kloner RA, Kostis JB. The second Princeton consensus on sexual dysfunction and cardiac risk: new guidelines for sexual medicine. *J Sex Med* 2006;3:28–36.

2. Safarinejad MR, Hosseini SY. Erectile dysfunction: clinical guidelines (1). *Urol J* 2004;1:133–147.

3. Foley S, Wittmann D, Balon R. A multidisciplinary approach to sexual dysfunction in medical education. *Acad Psychiatry* 2010;34:386–389.

4. Gall H et al. [Erectile dysfunction: a multidisciplinary approach]. *Z Hautkr* 1987;62:1145–1146, 1149–1150.

5. Kaiser FE et al. Impotence and aging: clinical and hormonal factors. *J Am Geriatr Soc* 1988;36:511–519.

6. Virag R, Bouilly P, Frydman D. Is impotence an arterial disorder? A study of arterial risk factors in 440 impotent men. *Lancet* 1985;1:181–184.

7. Williams T, Honeywell M, Branch III E, Ghazvini P, King K. Tadalafil in the treatment of erectile dysfunction. *Drug Forecast* 2004;29:295–303.

8. Stewart DJ, Pohl U, Bassange E. Free radicals inhibits endothelium-dependent dilation in the coronary resistance bed. *Am J Physiol* 1988;255:H765-H769.

9. Boger RH, Bode-Boger SM, Frolisch JC. The L-arginine-nitric oxide pathway: role in atherosclerosis and therapeutic implications. *Atherosclerosis* 1996;127:1–11.

10. Schwarz ER, Rastogi S, Rodriguez JJ, Kapur V, Sulemanjee N, Gupta R, Rosanio S. A multidisciplinary approach to assess erectile dysfunction in high-risk cardiovascular patients. *Int J Impot Res* 2005;17(Suppl 1):S37–43.

11. Dusing R. Sexual dysfunction in male patients with hypertension: influence of antihypertensive drugs. *Drugs* 2005;65:773–786.

12. Grimm HR, Grandits GA, Svendsen K, TOMHS Research Group. Incidence and disappearance of erectile problems in men treated with for stage I hypertension: the treatment of mild hypertension study (TOMHS). *Eur Urol* 1996;30(Suppl 2):26.

13. Silvestri A et al. Report of erectile dysfunction after therapy with beta blockers is related to patient knowledge of the side effects and is reversed by placebo. *Eur Heart J* 2003;24:1928–1932.

14. Croog SH, Levine S, Testa MA, Sudilovsky A. The effects on antihypertensive therapy on quality of life. *N Engl J Med* 1986;314:1657–1664.

15. Piha J, Kaaja R. Effects of monoxidine and metoprolol in penile circulation in hypertensive men with erectile dysfunction: results of a pilot study. *Int J Impot Res* 2003;5:287–289.

16. Ko DT et al. Beta-blocker therapy and symptoms of depression, fatigue, and sexual dysfunction. *JAMA* 2002;288:351–357.

17. Buffum J. Pharmosexology update: prescription drugs and sexual function. *J Psychoactive Drugs* 1986;18:97–106.

18. DiBianco R. A large-scale trial of captopril for mild to moderate heart failure in the primary care setting. *Clin Cardiol* 1991;14:676–682.

19. Fletcher SG, Castro-Borrero W, Remington G, Treadaway K, Lemack GE, Frohman EM. Sexual dysfunction in patients with multiple sclerosis: a multidisciplinary approach to evaluation and management. *Nat Clin Pract Urol* 2009;6:96–107.

20. McCabe MP. Exacerbation of symptoms among people with multiple sclerosis: impact on sexuality and relationships over time. *Arch Sex Behav* 2004;33:593–601.

21. Feldman HA, Longcope C, Derby C, Johannes C, Araujo AB, Coviello AD, Bremner WJ McKinlay JB. Age trends in the level of serum testosterone and other hormones in middle-aged men: longitudinal results from the Massachusetts Male Aging Study. *J Clin Endocrinol Metab* 2002;87:589–598.

22. Lakshman KM, Basaria S. Safety and efficacy of testosterone gel in the treatment of male hypogonadism. *Clin Interv Aging* 2009;4:397–412.

23. Araujo AB, O'Donnell AB, Brambilla DJ, Simpson WB, Longcope C, Matsumoto AM, McKinlay JB. Prevalence and incidence of androgen deficiency in middle-aged and older men: estimates from the Massachusetts Male Aging Study. *J Clin Endocrinol Metab* 2004;89:5920–5926.

24. Nickel JC, Morales A, Condra M, Fenemore J, Surridge DH. Endocrine dysfunction in impotence: incidence, significance and cost-effective screening. *J Urol* 1984;130:40–45.

25. Boyle P, McGinn R, Maisonneuve P, La Vecchia C. Epidemiology of benign prostatic hyperplasia: present knowledge and studies needed. *Eur Urol* 1991;20(suppl):3–9.

26. Sarica K et al. Multidisciplinary evaluation of diabetic impotence. *Eur Urol* 1994;26:314–318.

27. Jacobs JA et al. A multidisciplinary approach to the evaluation and management of male sexual dysfunction. *J Urol* 1983;129:35–38.

28. Montorsi F et al. Summary of the recommendations on sexual dysfunctions in men. *J Sex Med* 2010;7:3572–3588.

29. Lue TF et al. Summary of the recommendations on sexual dysfunctions in men. *J Sex Med* 2004;1:6–23.

30. Zamboni BD. The role of sex therapist in treating erectile dysfunction: Working toward multidisciplinary treatment with physicians. *Current Sexual Health Report* 2006;3:154–157.

31. Fink HA et al. Sildenafil for male erectile dysfunction. A systematic review and meta-analysis. *Arch Intern Med* 2002;162:1349–1360.

32. Porst H et al. The efficacy and tolerability of vardenafil, a new, oral, selective phosphodiesterase type 5 inhibitor, in patients with erectile dysfunction: the first at-home clinical trial. *Int J Impot Res* 2001;13:192–199.

33. Porst H, Padma-Nathan H, Giuliano F, Anglin G. Efficacy of tadalafil for the treatment of erectile dysfunction at 24 and 36 hours after dosing: a randomized controlled trial. *Urology* 2003;62:121–125.

34. Kloner RA. Cardiovascular effects of the 3 phosphodiesterase-5 inhibitors approved for the treatment of erectile dysfunction. *Circulation* 2004;110:3149–3155.

35. Safarinejad MR, Hosseini SY. Erectile dysfunction: clinical guidelines (2). *Urol J* 2004;1:227–239.

36. Dula E, Bukofzer S, Perdok R, George M, for the Apomorphine SL Study Group. Double-blind, crossover comparison on 3 mg apomorphine SL with placebo and with 4 mg apomorphine SL in male erectile dysfunction. *Eur Urol* 2001;39:558–563.

37. Guay AT et al. Yohimbine treatment of organic erectile dysfunction in a dose-escalation trial. *Int J Impot Res* 2002;14:25–31.

38. Morgentaler A. Male impotence. *Lancet* 1999;354:1713–1718.

39. Yamamoto S et al. The effects of replacing dihydropyridine calcium-channel blockers with angiotensin II receptor blocker on the quality of life in hypertensive patients. *Blood Pressure* 2003;12:22–28.

40. Meinhardt W, Schmitz Pl, Kropman RF, de la Fuente RB, Lycklama a Nijeholt AA, Zwartendijk J. Trazodone, a double blind trial for treatment of erectile dysfunction. *Int J Impot Res* 1997;9:163–165.

41. Safarinejad MR. Therapeutic effects of high-dose isoxsuprine in the management of mixed type impotence. *Urology* 2001;58:95–97.

42. Wang C et al. Long-term testosterone gel (AndroGel) treatment maintains beneficial effects on sexual function and mood, lean and fat mass, and bone mineral density in hypogonadal men. *J Clin Endocrinol Metab* 2004;89:2085–2098.

43. Virag R et al. Intracavernous self-injection of vasoactive drugs in the treatment of impotence: 8-year experience with 615 cases. *J Urol* 1991;145:287–292.

44. Vaidyanathan S, Krishnan KR. Myocardial infarction associated with intra-cavernosal administration of alprostadil in a patient with spinal cord injury and paraplegia. *Spinal Cord* 1996;34:754–755.

45. Bodner DR, Haas CA, Krueger B, Seftel AD. Intraurethral alprostadil for treatment of erectile dysfunction in patients with spinal cord injury. *Urology* 1999;53:199–202.

46. Porst H. Transurethral alprostadil with MUSE (medicated urethral system for erection) vs. intracavernous alprostadil: a comparative study in 103 patients with erectile dysfunction. *Int J Impot Res* 1997;9:187–192.

47. Lewis RW, Witherington R. External vacuum therapy for erectile dysfunction: use and results. *World J Urol* 1997;15:78–82.

48. Denil J, Ohl DA, Smythe C. Vacuum erection device in spinal cord injured men: patient and partner satisfaction. *Arch Phys Med Rehabil* 1996;77:750–753.

49. Levine LA, Estrada CR, Morgentaler A. Mechanical reliability and safety of and patient satisfaction with the Ambicor inflatable penile prosthesis: results of a 2 center study. *J Urol* 2001;166:932–937.

50. Carson CC, Mulcahy JJ, Govier FE, the AMS 700CX study group. Efficacy, safety and patient satisfaction outcomes of the AMS 700CX inflatable penile prosthesis: results of a longterm multicenter study. *J Urol* 2000;164:376–380.

51. American Psychiatric Association. *Diagnostic and Statistical manual, 4th Ed., text revision.* American Psychiatric Publishing Inc. Arlington, VA, 2000.

52. Laumann EO, Paik A, Rosen RC. Sexual dysfunction in the United States: prevalence and predictors. *JAMA* 1999;281(6):537–544.

53. Noonan RJ. Sex Surrogates: A Clarification of Their Functions Research Study, 1984. Available online at http://www.sexquest.com/surrogat.htm. Accessed on February 3, 2013.

54. Gurman AS and Jacobson NS. *The Clinical Handbook of Couples Therapy, third edition.* The Guilford Press. New York, NY, 2002.

55. Gabbard GO. *Textbook of Psychotherapeutic Treatments.* American Psychiatric Publishing Inc. Arlington, VA, 2009.

56. Engel GL. The clinical application of the biopsychosocial model. *Am J Psychiatry* 1980;137:535–544.

57. Solomon H, Man J, Martin E, Jackson G. Role of exercise treadmill testing in the management of erectile dysfunction: a joint cardiovascular/erectile dysfunction clinic. *Heart* 2003;89:671–672.

Chapter 8

Erectile Dysfunction: A Marker of Peripheral Vascular Disease?

Jason C. Huang and Brian H. Annex

With the vascular predominance of the anatomy of the penis, erectile dysfunction (ED) has long been thought to be associated with peripheral vascular disease. There was no surprise when it was found that ED occurred at a higher frequency among individuals with known heart and cerebrovascular disease. The risk factors for coronary artery disease such as age, hyperlipidemia, smoking, and diabetes have been tied to an increased risk of ED (1). While the process of maintaining an erection is multifactorial, involving proper nerve signaling and mental health in addition to vascular function, the majority of ED cases have been associated with a vascular etiology. In the past two decades, there has been increasing research into the pathophysiology of ED. While investigating the utility of phosphodiesterase inhibitors in the setting of angina, the noted improvement in ED was a breakthrough linking the etiology of vascular disease with ED. From that point, it has become increasingly clear that the utility of diagnosing ED extends beyond the realm of sexual health. An estimated 52% of men between 40 and 70 years of age have this medical issue (2). In the aging male population, early recognition of ED in the primary care setting may pay dividends as an additional marker for systemic vascular health.

ED is a form of vascular injury that despite extensive, direct-to-the-public advertising is often left out of the conversation when physicians discuss measures of systemic vascular insults such as ischemic heart disease, peripheral claudication, or cerebrovascular accident. Production of a proper penile erection is a complex coordination of vascular events initiated by helical artery dilation leading to an influx of blood flow into the corpora cavernosa. The "artery size hypothesis" posed by Montorsi and colleagues (3) poses potential relevance in the early identification of ED. The helical penile artery is the smallest in diameter in comparison to the coronary, internal carotid, and femoral arteries. Gradual atherosclerotic progression is typically the cause of angina in chronic coronary artery disease and claudication symptoms in the femoral arteries. With regard to ED, a progression of luminal obstruction in the penile artery would appear to be a significant limiting factor. If atherosclerosis does progress at a similar rate without preference for specific arterial vessels, ED should precede many cases of progressive vascular disease in the general population.

If the "artery size hypothesis" does indeed hold true, regular surveillance for ED in the primary care field among the aging male population becomes a topic as important as the likes of exertional dyspnea or angina. Increasing age, a family history of coronary artery disease (CAD), hypertension, tobacco use, and dyslipidemia all are well-known risk factors for CAD. Interventions with a proven mortality benefit in the setting of known CAD abound. A daily aspirin, improved cholesterol/blood pressure control, and lifestyle modifications, including diet and exercise, are just the start. The decision to send a patient for stress testing, carotid ultrasound, or ankle–brachial index assessment can be swayed by a compilation of his known risk factors. Use of the International Index of Erectile Function (IIEF), a validated questionnaire, or even a direct yes/no question about ED would be another tool that can identify the need for more aggressive evaluation of vascular disease. Given the time constraints of the primary care physician responsible for the preventive health measures of a continually aging patient population, this will represent an opportunity to review the available scientific evidence behind this theory that ED truly precedes a significant proportion of cases of vascular disease.

Peripheral vascular disease (PVD) has been long underdiagnosed and has not been well recognized in the medical community, but its prevalence is estimated to be 8 to 12 million individuals in the United States. It is often associated with the presence of peripheral artery disease, with or without classic claudication (leg pain on walking that is relieved with rest) symptoms. The PARTNERS program, a multicenter study in 350 primary care practices in the United States, compiled 6,979 patients who were either 70 years or older or between the ages of 50 and 69 with a prior history of tobacco use and/or diabetes. This study in 2001 (4) revealed that 29% of these patients had PVD. Of all these patients with PVD, 44% were newly diagnosed by an ankle–brachial index of 0.9 or less during the screening of patients with no prior history of PVD. This high proportion of undiagnosed patients was attributed to the atypical presentation of the majority of these patients with PVD. Only 10.1% of the individuals found to have PVD during this study presented with the classic claudication symptoms of PVD (exercise-induced calf pain that is elicited by exertion and resolves with rest); 30.8% of those identified with PVD during this study actually had no complaints of leg pain.

Few large studies are available identifying the association between ED and PVD. A study by Polonsky and colleagues in 2009 (5) screened for PVD by the ankle–brachial index in 690 men without a prior history of known vascular disease who had been referred for cardiac stress testing. This prior history was identified by a past history of myocardial infarction, coronary revascularization, or any known PVD, including prior revascularization, abnormal ankle–brachial index, or known vascular disease per the patient. Overall, 23% of these patients were identified with PVD, while 66% of these individuals with PVD were considered asymptomatic. Three hundred eleven men (45% overall) were found to have ED determined by the IIEF survey. Most notably, ED doubled this patient population's risk of having PVD from 16% to 32%. ED severity, identified as mild, moderate, or severe by the IIEF, also exhibited a significant correlation in risk for PVD, from 28% to 33% to 40%, respectively. In fact, by multivariate regression analysis, ED was found to be an independent predictor of PVD in addition to diabetes, tobacco use, and CAD.

If all PVD cases were symptomatic, then using PVD symptoms would be logical. However, the identification of PVD in the primary care setting is limited by the atypical symptomatic presentation of the vast majority of patients. In particular, some may question whether the approximately 31% of asymptomatic individuals with PVD (4) would require further intervention given their lack of leg pain. Yet, PVD identified by the ankle–brachial index has in itself been independently associated with a 30% 5-year risk of myocardial infarction, stroke, and vascular death (6). Aggressive identification and management of cardiovascular risk factors such as tobacco use, dyslipidemia, diabetes mellitus, and hypertension would thus be warranted.

Limited studies have also been reported with regard to the link between the frequency of cases of cerebrovascular accident, another form of PVD, and ED. A retrospective case-control study by Chung and colleagues (7) identified 1,501 patients with ED and compared the incidence of subsequent stroke over a 5-year period in comparison to 7,505 randomly selected individuals from Taiwan's Longitudinal Health Insurance Database, a randomly derived database of 1 million individuals from the 25.68 million citizens covered by Taiwan's National Health Insurance program. Excluded patients included those with a prior history of cerebrovascular accident or cardiovascular disease. Over the 5-year period, 12.5% of the patients with ED had a cerebrovascular accident as opposed to 9.7% of the general population. This difference remained statistically significant when adjusted for a prior history of hypertension, diabetes, CAD, and PVD as well as hyperlipidemia, thus strengthening the link between PVD and ED.

In conjunction, an 8-year longitudinal population-based cohort study from the Netherlands published by Schouten and colleagues (8) surveyed the roughly 28,000 inhabitants of the city of Krimpen. The researchers identified 1,248 men between the age of 50 to 75 who had no prior history of myocardial infarction, stroke, or abdominal aortic aneurysm and who were not taking a daily aspirin or nitrate. ED was then assessed within this population, with 22.8% having reduced erectile rigidity and another 8.7% exhibiting severe ED. Both the presence and the severity of ED significantly increased the risk of cardiovascular events in this study, identified by stroke, myocardial infarction, or sudden death with no other identified etiology, over an average follow-up period of 6.3 years. This significant increase in risk remained true after adjustment for dyslipidemia, hypertension, diabetes, and tobacco use.

In addition to cerebrovascular disease and PVD, strong interest lies in the relationship between CAD and ED. Limited data, as shown above, have found an increased frequency of PVD and stroke in patients with ED. It is well established that ED occurs at increased frequencies in patients with known CAD; it actually has been estimated to occur in 42% to 75% of patients with CAD (3) and 76% to 89% of patients with heart failure (9). The key issue, however, is whether ED precedes the development of symptomatic cardiovascular disease. Asymptomatic cardiovascular disease is typically identified by an assessment of a patient's known risk factors and subsequent stress testing if warranted. Awareness of ED in the middle-aged man could be another tool in the attempt to address the highest cause of mortality in the general male population today.

The prevalence of CAD in patients without a history of angina or myocardial infarction has ranged between 1.34% and 4.5% in older studies (10). In a limited prospective study (11) of patients with ED of vascular origin confirmed by Doppler ultrasound and no prior history of CAD, 50 men underwent exercise treadmill stress testing and stress echocardiography to identify asymptomatic CAD. A positive test was followed by coronary angiography. Interestingly, 19% of the study's patients were found to have significant CAD with at least 50% occlusion of any of the three coronary arteries. While the study population was small, there is the suggestion that the presence of ED can increase the risk of asymptomatic CAD by 5- to 10-fold.

In a prospective study, Gazzaruso and colleagues (12) identified 291 men with type 2 diabetes who had asymptomatic CAD. CAD was identified by angiography in those with a highly positive exercise ECG test or exercise stress thallium scintigraphy in those with a positive exercise ECG test or a positive dipyridamole stress test. These patients were followed for an average of 4 years while adverse cardiac events were recorded, including myocardial infarction, unstable angina, stroke/transient ischemic attack, symptomatic peripheral vascular disease, repeat revascularization, or death attributed to coronary artery disease or congestive heart failure. One hundred eighteen of the 291 patients (~40%) were found to have ED during the course of the study. Of this subset, 25% of the patients with ED had an adverse cardiac event over the course of the study as opposed to 11% of the patients without ED ($p = .001$). Thus, ED was found to be an independent risk factor that doubled the risk of a cardiac event in type 2 diabetic patients, who are already a group of patients with an increased risk for having a cardiac event.

Much of the literature reviewed thus far has been limited by a lack of large prospective studies relating the incidence of vascular disease to that of ED. One recent publication by Batty and colleagues (13) based on the ADVANCE trial (Action in Diabetes and Vascular Disease: Preterax and Diamicron Modified-Release Controlled Evaluation) followed 6,304 men aged 55 to 88 years with type 2 diabetes for 5 years while following outcomes such as the incidence of cardiovascular and cerebrovascular disease. These patients were obtained from an expansive study involving 215 centers from 20 countries identifying patients with type 2 diabetes and at least one additional risk factor for cardiovascular disease. Roughly half (3,158 of the 6,304) of the patients were found to have ED. In comparing the patient populations with and without ED at the start of this study, ED was associated with worse control over the typical risk factors associated with cardiovascular disease. This included statistically significant correlations with age, hemoglobin A1C, Body Mass Index, systolic blood pressure, serum creatinine, duration of diabetes, levels of inactivity measured by exercise episodes per week, and history of major macrovascular/microvascular disease, including stroke, myocardial infarction, macroalbuminuria, or diabetic retinopathy.

In a compilation of data over the 5-year study, patients with ED were found to have an increased risk of total mortality, cardiovascular disease, CAD, and cerebrovascular disease after adjustment for age and prior illnesses (13). Most notably, a 42% increase in risk of CAD was noted for patients with baseline ED. Over the course of the study, most of the patients were queried about symptoms of ED at the start of the study and 2 years into follow-up. In comparison to the patients without ED over the initial 2 years of the study, the patients who had ED at baseline exhibited statistically significant risk across the board, including total mortality, cardiovascular disease, coronary heart disease, cerebrovascular disease, dementia, and cognitive decline. In comparison, the patients who developed ED over the initial 2 years of the study exhibited an increased risk of only dementia. This variability between individuals with a baseline history of ED versus new-onset ED over the course of this 5-year study is substantial. There would appear to be a window for aggressive risk-factor modification in patients with recent-onset ED to limit significant endpoints such as overall mortality and incidence of stroke or myocardial infarction.

This finding is reinforced by one other large prospective, randomized controlled trial based on the Prostate Cancer Prevention Trial. This study, by Thompson and colleagues (14), evaluated 9,457 men aged 55 years or older who had been placed in the placebo arm of the Prostate Cancer Prevention Trial, which was designed to compare the benefit of finasteride over a 7-year period in patients with no prior history of prostate cancer and a normal prostate specific antigen level. This study focused on the 4,247 patients of the control arm who had no known prior history of cardiovascular disease or ED at the start. Over the 7-year course of this study, 65% of these patients reported incident ED. These patients exhibited a correlation between time after initial incident of ED and risk of an initial cardiovascular event, whether it be angina, myocardial infarction, stroke, arrhythmia, or congestive heart failure. In comparison between 1 year and 5 years after the initial ED incident, the prevalence of an initial cardiovascular event increased from 2% to 11%. In evaluating the patients who experienced a cardiovascular event during this study, incident ED was found to be a statistically significant risk factor in addition to the typical risk factors, including age, Body Mass Index, systolic blood pressure, HDL cholesterol, tobacco use, family history of myocardial infarction, and diabetes mellitus.

The association between ED and systemic vascular disease is becoming increasingly well established. The coordination of events involved in penile tumescence depends on an array of vascular components. The physiological etiology linking ED and vascular disease, however, remains complex and not completely understood. The "artery size hypothesis" (3) relies on a theory of a uniform increase in systemic atherosclerosis in the human body. Its explanation is based on an idea of increasing vascular obstruction leading to limited filling of the corpora cavernosa. This mechanism would thus predict a chronological occurrence of ED prior to coronary disease as well as cerebrovascular disease. Yet the occurrence of CAD is more complex than a gradual progression of obstructive atherosclerosis. It has been well established that acute myocardial infarction typically occurs in the setting of atherosclerotic plaque rupture leading to activation of the clotting cascade and subsequent coronary vessel obstruction. Instead of the steady progression of atherosclerosis leading to pure luminal obstruction, endothelial cell dysfunction is a phenomenon believed to precede the initial development of atherosclerosis and subsequent CAD. In conjunction, endothelial dysfunction has been implicated as the common denominator in systemic vascular disease.

Endothelial cell dysfunction is a cornerstone of both the risk for atherosclerosis as well as a potentiating disease by making the endothelial wall more prone to injury and eventual atherosclerosis (15). As the barrier between blood and tissue, the vascular endothelium serves multiple purposes as a selectively permeable gateway as well as a signaling center for control of vascular tone. The endothelial cells themselves are able to influence the surrounding vascular smooth muscle with an array of signaling factors, including vasoconstrictors such as angiotensin II and vasodilators such as prostacyclin and nitric oxide. The proper regulation of blood flow thus becomes a complex coordination of vasoconstriction and vasodilation that can be disrupted by insults to any of the complex signaling pathways of the vascular system.

Since the discovery of the utility of phosphodiesterase (PDE) inhibitors in the treatment of ED, nitric oxide-dependent vasodilation has been a point of emphasis in research into further therapeutic options for ED. The direct effect of PDE inhibitors in the physiology of the vascular endothelium is an obstruction of the PDE-5 enzyme in the surrounding vascular smooth muscle cells (16). This enzyme is normally involved in the breakdown of cyclic guanosine monophosphate (cGMP), which induces vascular smooth muscle cell relaxation by lowering the concentration of intracellular calcium. Proper maintenance of cGMP levels is thus crucial in the coordination of smooth muscle tone in the maintenance of blood flow through the vascular system. cGMP is produced by guanylate cyclase, an enzyme activated directly by nitric oxide. In the setting of endothelial dysfunction, the disruption of upstream signaling markers in the production of nitric oxide can offset the coordination of the chronological events involved in producing a penile erection.

The inhibition of the PDE-5 enzyme by PDE inhibitors concentrates cGMP activity, potentiating the effect of available nitric oxide produced by the endothelial cell. Vascular disease in the setting of ED appears to be a manifestation of sufficient endothelial dysfunction associated with insufficient nitric oxide production (17). While PDE inhibitors represent a popular and well-known medication in the treatment of ED, it has been estimated that approximately half of the men with ED experience no benefit from these medications. The reason for this large proportion remains unclear. One theory is that these patients have a level of endothelial dysfunction marked by a severe limitation of nitric oxide production. Given that PDE inhibitors potentiate the downstream effects of nitric oxide, there may be a threshold requiring a certain amount of nitric oxide production for the desired response to these medications.

Further research into the upstream mechanisms of proper signaling in endothelial function continues to develop. In addition to ED, this research is of significant interest in the realm of cardiovascular disease and PVD. Significant attention has been directed at a number of cytokine growth factors such as vascular endothelial cell growth factor, basic fibroblast growth factor, placenta growth factor, and angiopoietin (18). These signaling markers are being investigated as potential targets for genetic upregulation leading to a theoretical increase in surrounding angiogenesis and improved vascular perfusion. With growing evidence of benefit in animal models of ED (19), the development of therapeutic angiogenesis offers further evidence of the impact of vascular disease on ED.

Endothelial dysfunction has become increasingly evident as the underlying factor in systemic vascular disease, whether it be in the heart, peripheral perfusion, or penis. While new therapeutic options are being investigated for ED treatment, attention should be directed to the potential mortality benefit in aggressively treating men with new-onset ED for the many risk factors associated with cardiovascular disease. In addition, closer surveillance for other signs of PVD, CAD, or risk of cerebrovascular disease appears to be warranted. While the theory of increasing atherosclerosis behind the "artery size hypothesis" does not appear to be the true etiology of ED, the vessels responsible for a proper penile erection are likely more sensitive to gradually increasing endothelial dysfunction given the smaller vessel diameter in comparison to the coronary or carotid vessels. The available evidence does suggest that ED is associated with an increased incidence of PVD, stroke, and cardiovascular events. More importantly, the patients with new-onset ED in the available studies do not exhibit the same risk as the patients with longstanding ED. Early recognition of this prevalent issue in the aging male patient thus holds significant benefit in the treatment of the overall health of this population.

References

1. Fung MM, Bettencourt R, Barrett-Connor E. Heart disease risk factors predict erectile dysfunction 25 years later: the Rancho Bernardo Study. *J Am Coll Cardiol* 2004;43(8):1405–1411.

2. Feldman HA, Goldstein I, Hatzichristou DG, Krane RJ, McKinlay JB. Impotence and its medical and psychosocial correlates: results of the Massachusetts Male Aging Study. *J Urol* 1994;151(1):54–61.

3. Montorsi P, Ravagnani PM, Galli S, et al. The artery size hypothesis: a macrovascular link between erectile dysfunction and coronary artery disease. *Am J Cardiol* 2005;96(12B):19M-23M.

4. Hirsch AT, Criqui MH, Treat-Jacobson D, et al. Peripheral arterial disease detection, awareness, and treatment in primary care. *JAMA* 2001;286(11):1317–1324.

5. Polonsky TS, Taillon LA, Sheth H, Min JK, Archer SL, Ward RP. The association between erectile dysfunction and peripheral arterial disease as determined by screening ankle-brachial index testing. *Atherosclerosis* 2009;207(2):440–444.

6. Newman AB, Shemanski L, Manolio TA, et al. Ankle-arm index as a predictor of cardiovascular disease and mortality in the Cardiovascular Health Study. The Cardiovascular Health Study Group. *Arterioscler Thromb Vasc Biol* 1999;19(3):538–545.

7. Chung SD, Chen YK, Lin HC, Lin HC. Increased risk of stroke among men with erectile dysfunction: a nationwide population-based study. *J Sex Med* 2011;8(1):240–246.

8. Schouten BW, Bohnen AM, Bosch JL, et al. Erectile dysfunction prospectively associated with cardiovascular disease in the Dutch general population: results from the Krimpen Study. *Int J Impot Res* 2008;20(1):92–99.

9. Hebert K, Lopez B, Macedo FY, Gomes CR, Urena J, Arcement LM. Peripheral vascular disease and erectile dysfunction as predictors of mortality in heart failure patients. *J Sex Med* 2009;6(7):1999–2007.

10. Enbergs A, Burger R, Reinecke H, Borggrefe M, Breithardt G, Kerber S. Prevalence of coronary artery disease in a general population without suspicion of coronary artery disease: angiographic analysis of subjects aged 40 to 70 years referred for catheter ablation therapy. *Eur Heart J* 2000;21(1):45–52.

11. Vlachopoulos C, Rokkas K, Ioakeimidis N, et al. Prevalence of asymptomatic coronary artery disease in men with vasculogenic erectile dysfunction: a prospective angiographic study. *Eur Urol* 2005;48(6):996–1003.

12. Gazzaruso C, Solerte SB, Pujia A, et al. Erectile dysfunction as a predictor of cardiovascular events and death in diabetic patients with angiographically proven asymptomatic coronary artery disease: a potential protective role for statins and 5-phosphodiesterase inhibitors. *J Am Coll Cardiol* 2008;51(21):2040–2044.

13. Batty GD, Li Q, Czernichow S, et al. Erectile dysfunction and later cardiovascular disease in men with type 2 diabetes: prospective cohort study based on the ADVANCE (Action in Diabetes and Vascular Disease: Preterax and Diamicron Modified-Release Controlled Evaluation) trial. *J Am Coll Cardiol* 2010;56(23):1908–1913.

14. Thompson IM, Tangen CM, Goodman PJ, Probstfield JL, Moinpour CM, Coltman CA. Erectile dysfunction and subsequent cardiovascular disease. *JAMA* 2005;294(23):2996–3002.

15. Schwartz BG, Economides C, Mayeda GS, Burstein S, Kloner RA. The endothelial cell in health and disease: its function, dysfunction, measurement and therapy. *Int J Impot Res* 2010;22(2):77–90.

16. Goldstein I, Lue TF, Padma-Nathan H, Rosen RC, Steers WD, Wicker PA. Oral sildenafil in the treatment of erectile dysfunction. Sildenafil Study Group. *N Engl J Med* 1998;338(20):1397–1404.

17. Morelli A, Vignozzi L, Filippi S, Mancina R, Maggi M. Erectile dysfunction: molecular biology, pathophysiology and pharmacological treatment. *Minerva Urol Nefrol* 2005;57(2):85–90.

18. Maas R, Schwedhelm E, Albsmeier J, Boger RH. The pathophysiology of erectile dysfunction related to endothelial dysfunction and mediators of vascular function. *Vasc Med* 2002;7(3):213–225.

19. Yamanaka M, Shirai M, Shiina H, et al. Vascular endothelial growth factor restores erectile function through inhibition of apoptosis in diabetic rat penile crura. *J Urol* 2005;173(1):318–323.

Chapter 9

Chronic Diseases and ED After Organ Transplantation

Anita Phan and Ernst R. Schwarz

Introduction

The majority of published data on erectile dysfunction (ED) after organ transplantation is found in the renal transplant literature. The prevalence of, potential mechanisms of, and therapeutic options for ED have primarily been investigated and described in renal transplant patients, with limited studies on other solid organ transplant recipients such as heart and liver. Despite the studies published on ED after organ transplantation, the extent of knowledge in this field remains relatively limited.

Prevalence

The prevalence of ED is disproportionately elevated in those with chronic diseases, including renal insufficiency, liver dysfunction, and heart failure. Sexual dysfunction affects well over half of patients in the end stages of organ dysfunction. In chronic heart failure the prevalence of sexual dysfunction is as high as 84% in men (1), while 50% of patients with end-stage renal disease are affected (2, 3), with a prevalence among those on dialysis of over 80% (4–7). In contrast to the general population, where 31% of American men are affected by ED (8), those with chronic diseases reportedly have a higher prevalence. It could be hypothesized that being subject to a chronic disease, such as renal insufficiency, contributes to ED, and therefore organ transplantation would lead not only to resolution of the chronic disease but also reduction in the number of those affected by ED. However, in reality, ED continues to affect many patients even after organ transplantation.

Some of the neuroendocrine disturbances that contribute to ED in patients with end-stage renal disease are alleviated after kidney transplantation (9), although reports of ED remain as high as 55% to 75% of patients even after transplantation (10–14). Although the majority of published data support that after renal transplantation there is a decrease in the prevalence of those without sexual activity, an increase in sexual desire (15), and improvement in sexual functioning (2, 4, 6, 13, 15–24), there have been reports of continued and even worsened erectile or sexual functioning after kidney transplantation (5, 11, 15,

20, 22, 25, 26). In a longitudinal study conducted by Laupacis and colleagues, sexual dysfunction was the only symptom that did not significantly improve after kidney transplantation in hemodialysis patients (27). Sexual function in the organ transplant population has been regarded as an important aspect of quality of life (1, 18, 28), and interestingly, of the many quality-of-life measures, it is one of the measures that did not significantly improve after transplantation (27, 29, 30).

Kidney transplant recipients are not the only organ recipients who continue to be afflicted by ED. Despite improvements in cardiac function and decon-ditioning in patients with end-stage heart failure who have undergone heart transplantation, the prevalence of sexual dysfunction not only persists (29–33) but also remains a prominent issue, with as many as 78% of men affected by ED for years after transplantation (30). Sexual dysfunction in heart transplant recipients includes ED, ejaculation problems, and avoidance of sexual oppor-tunities (32). After heart transplantation, it did not appear that libido changed, while erectile rigidity and orgasmic ability worsened (29).

As many as 70% of patients with chronic liver disease are affected by ED (34). After liver transplantation, the prevalence of ED decreases, although 30% to 50% of recipients are still affected (35–37). In a study done by Ho and associates on patients with end-stage liver disease who received liver transplantation, 32% complained of *de novo* sexual dysfunction (37).

Quality of Life

Quality of life, as defined by the World Health Organization, encompasses phys-ical, psychological, and social domains, and improvement in all aspects occurs after organ transplantation. In general, quality of life significantly improves after organ transplantation, with multiple published reports in lung, heart, kidney, pancreas, and liver recipients (18). It has been reported that organ transplan-tation has a positive impact on sexuality, with no significant difference in sat-isfaction across different transplant groups with regard to sexual functioning and quality of life (38), but despite these reports, the prevalence of sexual dysfunction remains considerably elevated, indeed, over a quarter of transplant recipients being sexually inactive (38). Although the majority of studies on heart transplant recipients have reported an improvement in quality of life after transplantation (18, 39–42), those with sexual dysfunction have scored lower on quality-of-life questionnaires than those without sexual dysfunction (30). Components of quality-of-life questionnaires dealing with sexual life and sexual functioning, including sexual drive, interest, and performance, were found to be less favorably scored than other measures of quality of life (30, 43).

Etiology

The pathophysiology of sexual dysfunction after solid organ transplantation is multifactorial, including endocrine, anatomical, neurogenic, autonomic, phar-macological, and psychosocial factors. The predominance of any one of these factors as the primary cause for ED in the transplant recipient remains unclear.

Although organ transplant recipients are subject to the same predisposing factors for ED as the general population, such as age, hypertension, diabetes mellitus, and depression, additional factors specific to the transplant population also play a role, including neuroendocrine changes and immunosuppressive therapy. There are also factors specific to different organ transplants that may affect erectile function, including iterative transplants and the surgical approach used in kidney transplant recipients.

Age

Age is independently associated with ED in the general population and also plays a significant role in organ transplant recipients (11, 12, 14, 29, 35, 44). The impact of age in the transplant population appears to be more complex than that of the general population. The prevalence of sexual dysfunction is as high as 55.7% in kidney recipients, even though they were younger than a normal control group (11). A study performed by Pourmand and colleagues on 64 hemodialysis patients followed after transplantation found that younger age at the time of transplantation was significantly associated with improvement in erectile functioning (6). Studies have also demonstrated that ED after kidney transplantation was less severe in younger patients, and the younger recipients had more significant improvement than their older counterparts (4, 6).

In contrast to those findings, Mirone and colleagues reported that sexual functioning did not change in those older than 45 years of age and may actual worsen in younger recipients, with a decrease in their International Index of Erectile Function (IIEF) score after transplantation (5). This paradox of younger transplant recipients with more severe ED after transplantation may be secondary to psychological contributions, because they may have greater sexual expectations than their older counterparts (5).

Neuroendocrine System

Neuroendocrine hormones that affect sexual functioning are altered in end-stage organ disorders as well as after organ transplantation. The hypothalamic-pituitary-gonadal axis is altered in end-stage liver, kidney, and heart disease, influencing levels of sexual hormones including testosterone, prolactin, luteinizing hormone (LH), and follicle stimulating hormone (FSH) (23, 45, 46). In patients with end-stage liver disease, lower levels of total testosterone and elevated levels of prolactin and sex hormone binding globulin (SHBG) all improved after liver transplantation (46). Uremia in chronic renal disease affects gonadal function with hypospermatogenesis, infertility, and impotence, and was found to be reversed after kidney transplantation (9). Levels of prolactin and estradiol have also been found to return to normal limits after kidney transplantation (47).

Immunosuppressive therapy with the use of steroids influences the hypothalamic-pituitary-gonadal axis. In the early period after a heart transplant, patients have low serum testosterone levels along with elevated levels of LH and FSH, likely secondary to suppression of the hypothalamic-pituitary-gonadal axis from medications such as prednisone (48). The first year after heart transplantation, low levels of testosterone levels were found in 14% of recipients; they persisted in 18% after the second year (48). Although in the early posttransplantation period low testosterone levels may be due to secondary hypogonadism, in the later years the mechanism may actually be due to primary gonadal dysfunction, as evidenced by low testosterone levels in the setting of elevated gonadotropin levels (48). It is unclear whether steroids have an effect on ED, although there has been a report of decreased IIEF scores when compared to scores prior to transplantation (5).

Testosterone is important for the onset of erection, with low levels being correlated with sexual dysfunction in kidney transplantation (22). Despite these changes in neurohormonal levels before and after transplantation, their role in sexual functioning after transplantation remains to be elucidated. Some trials have demonstrated that kidney transplant recipients with normal serum levels of testosterone can still experience ED. Levels of sex hormones such as prolactin, LH, and FSH have not been found to be significantly different in renal transplant patients with and without ED (20). Immunosuppressive agents have been found to have specific effects on neurohormonal levels (see the section "Medications" later in this chapter).

Vascular

Vascular insufficiency is one of the reported causes of ED in patients with kidney transplantation. Over 50% of ED cases in renal transplant patients were attributed to vasculogenic impotence due to arterial insufficiency and veno-occlusive dysfunction (22). Vascular evaluation of impotent renal transplant recipients reported that arterial occlusive disease, as evidenced by color Doppler ultrasound, played a significant role in 42.9% of cases, while 68.6% of patients had veno-occlusive dysfunction and 22.9% had mixed arterial and veno-occlusive dysfunction (49).

Just as in the general population, comorbidities such as hypercholesterolemia, hypertension, and diabetes mellitus are associated with ED after transplantation (2, 49). Hypercholesterolemia may contribute to vascular pathologies by enhancement of lipid deposition and development of vasculogenic ED (49). These comorbidities may also act through a mechanism of endothelial dysfunction (50) by impairing nitric oxide release (51), interfering with smooth muscle relaxation. End-stage renal disease is associated with dysfunction in endothelial-dependent vasodilation, a problem that persists even after kidney transplantation (52). Heart transplant recipients, like kidney transplant recipients, also suffer from endothelial dysfunction (53), thereby placing them at risk for ED.

Vascular pathophysiology along with blood flow supply is an important aspect of erectile functioning. The majority of blood supply to the penis comes from branches off the internal iliac arteries, so the surgical approach used in the kidney transplant recipient may affect sexual functioning. Renal transplantation is primarily done with either end-to-end anastomosis of the internal iliac artery or end-to-side anastomosis to the external iliac artery. Some surgeons prefer using the internal iliac artery for anastomosis (54), creating a concern for ED due to decreased blood flow to the penis because its blood supply is derived from the internal iliac arteries. Some believe that the use of the internal iliac arteries for end-to-end anastomosis in kidney transplantation does not have a significant effect on erectile function (4, 14, 24), while others believe it can compromise penile arterial supply, leading to ED (4, 22, 49, 54).

A trial performed by Nghiem and colleagues on impotence after renal transplantation did not find the ankle–brachial index or the penile–brachial index to be correlated with impotence (55). It has been reported that ligation of both internal iliac arteries did not result in pelvic devascularization (55), although this remains a concern as other trials have observed that both patients with iterative kidney transplantation (11, 22, 54) and those with internal iliac artery interruption had a higher prevalence of ED among renal transplantation recipients (14, 49). Due to the potential for compromised penile blood flow based on the surgical approach, there have been recommendations to use end-to-side anastomosis of the graft to the external iliac artery in those with impaired pelvic blood flow to decrease the risk of ED (11, 24, 49).

Psychosocial

Many studies, including the Massachusetts Male Aging Study, demonstrated an association between sexual dysfunction and psychological factors such as depression and poor mental health in the general population (56–59). Psychosocial factors are often present in chronic disease states and have also been found to be related to sexual dysfunction (60), and they often persist after organ transplantation. A study performed on kidney transplant recipients found that in those with ED, 21% attributed it to nonorganic causes (22), with performance anxiety and fear of causing harm to the transplanted kidney playing important roles (14, 22). Heart transplant patients with ED have also expressed concerns about harming the transplanted heart (32).

Depression is associated with ED after kidney transplantation. In the renal transplant population, depression was significantly associated with ED, with close to 30% suffering from depression (12). In contrast, when liver transplant recipients were asked about the main factor contributing to sexual dysfunction, only 10% attributed it to depression (37). In heart transplant patients, the impact of mental health and depressive symptoms was not significantly different in those with and without sexual dysfunction, while impaired physical functioning and general health were correlated with sexual function (30). This may suggest that sexual dysfunction in these patients may be more influenced by physiological rather than psychological factors (30).

Physical Health

Both mental health and physical health have been correlated with sexual function in the transplant population (61). Although physical functioning improves after heart transplantation, those with sexual dysfunction had a worse perception of their physical functioning and limitations compared to those without sexual dysfunction (30). Similar findings have also been demonstrated in the renal transplant literature (61), with the physical aspects of health-related quality of life, such as bodily pain, general health, physical role, and vitality, being related to ED rather than the mental components (44). Physical functioning is an important aspect as it relates to sexual activity. A mismatch between sexual desire and sexual performance is described after heart transplantation, with strong or improved libido but persistent or impaired sexual functioning (29). After heart transplants, patients with sexual dysfunction have significantly worse physical health, including physical functioning and physical role limitations, than their counterparts without sexual dysfunction (30).

Medications

When liver transplant recipients were asked about the main factor contributing to their sexual dysfunction, about one third believed it was medication-induced (37). Multiple medications have been implicated in sexual dysfunction with effects on libido, spermatogenesis, hormones, and erectile function. Organ transplant recipients face the added complications of taking immunosuppressive therapy, with medication regimens that may not only have interactions with other drugs, but also have direct physiological effects on sexual functioning.

Immunosuppressive therapy in the transplant population usually comprises triple therapy with corticosteroids, calcineurin inhibitors, and an antiproliferative agent. The effects of corticosteroids on sexual functioning and hormones were described in the "Neuroendocrine" section of this chapter. Cyclosporine is a calcineurin inhibitor widely used as part of immunosuppressive therapy. Animal studies performed on the effects of cyclosporine have demonstrated potential adverse effects on sexual functioning, including gonadotoxicity with decreased spermatogenesis and inhibition of testicular synthesis of testosterone despite elevation in LH levels (62, 63). Animal studies not only demonstrated direct Leydig cell effects of cyclosporine with decreased biosynthesis of testosterone (62–64) but also reveal central effects with suppression of the hypothalamic-pituitary-gonadal axis resulting in decreases in LH production and testosterone levels (65).

Endothelial functioning is another important aspect of normal erectile functioning, and cyclosporine has been demonstrated to have an effect on nitric oxide and smooth muscle dilation (66). In animal studies, cyclosporine inhibits smooth muscle relaxation, with reduction of nitric oxide metabolites leading to endothelial dysfunction (67, 68). It also has a pro-apoptotic effect, altering the extracellular matrix by increasing collagen formation (69). Chronic use of cyclosporine has been reported to be associated with fibrosis, as seen with cyclosporine-induced nephrotoxicity, and it could be postulated that similar effects occur in the corpora cavernosa, although animal studies of chronic exposure to cyclosporine have not yet demonstrated a direct influence on the function of erectile tissue (70).

In human studies, the effect of immunosuppressive therapy on sexual hormones and their relation to sexual functioning remains unclear. After renal transplantation, patients taking immunosuppressive therapy with calcineurin inhibitors, including both sirolimus and tacrolimus, were not found to have significantly different levels of LH and FSH compared to pretransplant levels (23, 71, 72). The effects of cyclosporine on testosterone levels appear to vary: some trials showed no significant change in levels (71), while others showed a significant increase (23). These differences in testosterone levels may be related to the timing of sampling, as testosterone levels are initially low after transplantation and return to normal levels even when the patient is taking cyclosporine (47, 48, 73). A trial performed on heart transplant recipients demonstrated that testosterone levels were lowest after the first month after the transplant and eventually normalized (48). Similar to animal studies, the mechanism of decreased serum testosterone in transplant patients may be due to both primary and secondary hypogonadism (48). After heart transplantation, recipients have been found to have low testosterone levels, along with low levels of FSH and LH, regardless of their immunosuppressive regimen, suggesting that the hypothalamic-pituitary-gonadal axis is impaired (74). Direct effects on gonadal function from immunosuppressants may also be present, as these patients do not respond to human chorionic gonadotropin administration (74).

It remains unclear how hormonal changes influenced by calcineurin inhibitors affect sexual functioning in organ transplant recipients. The effects of cyclosporine-based immunosuppressive therapy on ED remain controversial: some studies show a significant association with ED (5, 14, 20), while others could not demonstrate such an association (11, 75). The effects of calcineurin inhibitors on endothelial functioning and ED in humans remain to be established; thus far, no association has been demonstrated (13, 76).

Sirolimus, a rapamycin inhibitor, is used as an antiproliferative agent in immunosuppressive therapies. The use of sirolimus in both kidney and heart transplant patients is associated with lower levels of total testosterone and significantly elevated levels of LH, FSH, and SHBG (77–79), with the duration of treatment being correlated with the different levels of gonadotropins (78). Rapamycin inhibitors, such as sirolimus and everolimus, also have harmful effects on the testis and gonadal function, with disruption in spermatogenesis (79). A retrospective trial on kidney transplant patients taking sirolimus with and without calcineurin inhibitors found testosterone levels to be significantly lower in the patients taking sirolimus without calcineurin inhibitors (80). The group with the highest level of testosterone was the one taking calcineurin inhibitors without sirolimus (80), leading to the conclusion that sirolimus does in fact impair gonadal function after transplantation. Despite the hormonal changes and gonadal impact of rapamycin inhibitors, sirolimus-based therapies have not been associated with sexual dysfunction or ED (14, 77), and their clinical impact remains to be determined.

Immunosuppressive agents are not the only medications that may affect sexual functioning in transplant recipients. Both patients with kidney and heart transplants often have comorbidities and receive medical therapy that affect sexual functioning. Many transplant recipients have hypertension or develop hypertension due to immunosuppressive therapy, and they are subject to the same side effects from antihypertensives as the general population. Antihypertensives such as beta-adrenoreceptor blockers, alpha blockers, and diuretics have all been shown to contribute to ED (5, 13, 81–85). The effects of beta-adrenoreceptor blockers on sexual dysfunction have been well established. A comparison between atenolol and valsartan showed that atenolol decreased sexual activity and lowered testosterone levels, while valsartan increased sexual activity with no effect on testosterone levels (84). Angiotensin receptor blockers have also been implicated in sexual dysfunction in liver transplant recipients (35). Other medications, such as statins for those with concomitant hypercholesterolemia, may also play a role in ED (83).

Treatment

Treatment options for ED in the transplant population are similar to those for the general population, although factors such as drug interactions and infection risks need to be kept in mind. Transplant patients who seek treatment for their sexual dysfunction have a high rate of response (86). Eighty percent of renal transplant patients with ED who underwent some method of therapy reported a positive response (87).

Phosphodiesterase Type 5 Inhibitors

Phosphodiesterase type 5 (PDE-5) inhibitors, intracavernosal injections of alprostadil, testosterone therapy, and penile prostheses have all been used in the transplant population (88, 89).

Sildenafil, a PDE-5 inhibitor, acts by inhibiting cyclic guanosine monophosphate and is by far the best-studied therapeutic intervention for ED in the organ transplant population. Sildenafil, like immunosuppressive agents such as cyclosporine and tacrolimus, is metabolized through cytochrome P-450 enzymes, and therefore concern may be raised about the concomitant use of this drug with immunosuppressive agents or those metabolized through the same pathway. In the transplant population clinicians must take into account appropriate immunosuppressive levels in the blood and drug–drug interactions. The use of sildenafil in conjunction with cyclosporine has not been found to have a significant effect on the concentration of cyclosporine in the blood (26, 86, 90). Sildenafil used in conjunction with tacrolimus also did not prove to have any significant interaction with tacrolimus levels or pharmacokinetics (91–93).

The vast majority of trials on sildenafil in kidney transplant recipients taking immunosuppressive therapy have demonstrated both efficacy and safety (26, 86, 90, 91, 94). In the renal transplant population, sildenafil significantly improved all domains of sexual functioning, including ED, with the exception of sexual desire (86, 90, 91). In the transplant population, a sildenafil dose of 50 mg (86, 90) was found to be more effective than 25 mg or 100 mg (26, 87). Reported side effects of sildenafil in transplant recipients were similar to those in the general population and included facial flushing (93, 95), headache (26, 93–95), nasal congestion (93, 94), seasickness (94), gastric disorder (93), and visual disturbances (87). Overall, sildenafil was found to be safe, with few side effects, in the transplant population (86, 90).

Sildenafil also acts as a vasodilator and can result in systemic vasodilation. Although sildenafil did not affect the pharmacokinetics or levels of tacrolimus, tacrolimus may affect the pharmacokinetics of sildenafil, leading to a decrease in systemic blood pressure (93, 95). Caution would therefore be needed to prevent systemic hypotension, although heart transplant recipients using sildenafil did not demonstrate hypotension despite concomitant use of their usual antihypertensive medications (96, 97). A trial performed by Malavaud and colleagues on the glomerular filtration rate of kidney transplant patients taking sildenafil found that it did not impair renal graft function; rather, patients had a transient increase in the glomerular filtration rate (95).

Sildenafil was demonstrated to be effective not only in kidney transplant patients but also in heart and liver transplant patients (37, 96, 97). Compared to the kidney transplant literature, PDE-5 inhibitors have not been as well studied in other solid organ transplant populations for the treatment of ED, although the data available suggest similar safety and efficacy after transplantation (37, 96, 97).

Vardenafil, another PDE-5 inhibitor, has been shown to have similar beneficial effects as sildenafil on ED in renal transplant patients, with improvement in scores on the IIEF, safety with concomitant use of cyclosporine and tacrolimus, and minimal side effects (98). Side effects with vardenafil were found in 18% of users (headaches, palpitations, flushing, and dyspepsia) (98). Levels of sex hormones, including LH, FSH, prolactin, and testosterone, were not significantly affected by vardenafil (98).

Prostaglandin E1

Intracavernosal injection of vasoactive drugs such as prostaglandin E1 is also beneficial in the treatment of ED in the transplant population (87, 99). Studies on the efficacy and safety of prostaglandin E1 have been reported in both the kidney (87, 99) and heart transplant (100) populations. In a study performed on renal transplant recipients treated for ED, those who failed to respond to sildenafil therapy tried intracavernosal injections, with good response (87). Eighty percent of those using this method of treatment had good erections and complete satisfaction, with no systemic complications (87). Intracavernosal injections of prostaglandin E1 has been reported to be successful in 90% of those who have employed this method, with no adverse local or systemic complications aside from local pain at the injection site (99). Heart transplant patients with organic impotence demonstrated similar results as kidney transplant patients, with no significant side effects (100). Aside from local pain at the injection site (100), there were no reports of priapism (87) or alteration in immunosuppressant levels, including cyclosporine and azathioprine (99).

Penile Prosthesis

The use of a penile prosthesis as a treatment for ED is controversial in organ transplant recipients due to their immunocompromised state and concern for increased risk of infection. In general, a penile prosthesis has been viewed as the last option for vasculogenic ED. A study performed by Sidi and colleagues on diabetic patients with organ transplantation found that a penile prosthesis as treatment for organic impotence did not cause any infections or erosion complications (101). Studies performed on heart and kidney transplant recipients also found successful implantation of a penile prosthesis, with no problems related to the prosthesis or infection (87, 102, 103). The timing of the prosthesis implantation may also be a factor in the rate of infectious complications. A retrospective study performed in renal transplant patients with a penile prosthesis found that those who had their prosthesis placed after transplantation did not have any complications for up to 40 months, while those who received the penile prosthesis prior to transplantation had infectious complications (5).

The use of a penile prosthesis in the transplant population appears to be an efficacious option, although reports of life-threatening infection have been published, and therefore careful consideration is warranted (104). Complications other than infections include malfunction of the device. A retrospective study performed on all penile prosthesis placed by one urologist at one institution found that kidney and pancreas transplant recipients had a 22% rate of complications with the penile prosthesis, compared to close to 8% in the nontransplant group (105). The rate of infection was similar in both groups with similar cultured organisms, although the rate of malfunction was higher in the transplant population, with autoinflation accounting for the difference in complication rates, with all malfunction complications occurring in patients who received the three-piece prosthesis (105).

Other Treatments

Other methods used for the treatment of ED includes testosterone treatment, although there are only very limited data showing that after transplantation there may be improvement in sexual dysfunction with hormone replacement therapy (87). Psychosexual therapy has also been employed in transplant patients with some efficacy and can be an important complement to pharmacological and surgical options (87).

Conclusion

Sexual functioning is an important aspect of quality of life that is often overlooked in the transplant population. Despite the high prevalence of ED and the gaps of knowledge in sexual functioning after organ transplantation, more than three quarters of organ recipients received no instructions concerning sexuality or fertility (38). The effects of organ transplantation on sexual function and ED remain controversial, with further investigation needed to elucidate etiological factors and therapeutic options. Although further studies will need to be done to provide improved therapeutic options, it must be kept in mind that current therapies have demonstrated positive effects in the treatment of ED, but these cannot be offered if the issue is not addressed.

References

1. Schwarz ER, Kapur V, Bionat S, Rastogi S, Gupta R, Rosanio S. The prevalence and clinical relevance of sexual dysfunction in women and men with chronic heart failure. *Int J Impot Res* 2008;20(1):85–91.

2. Barroso LV, Miranda EP, Cruz NI, et al. Analysis of sexual function in kidney transplanted men. *Transplant Proc* 2008;40(10):3489–3491.

3. Rodger RS, Fletcher K, Dewar JH, et al. Prevalence and pathogenesis of impotence in one hundred uremic men. *Uremia Invest* 1984;8(2):89–96.

4. Mehrsai A, Mousavi S, Nikoobakht M, Khanlarpoor T, Shekarpour L, Pourmand G. Improvement of erectile dysfunction after kidney transplantation: the role of the associated factors. *Urol J* 2006;3(4):240–244.

5. Mirone V, Longo N, Fusco F, et al. Renal transplantation does not improve erectile function in hemodialysed patients. *Eur Urol* 2009;56(6):1047–1053.

6. Pourmand G, Emamzadeh A, Moosavi S, et al. Does renal transplantation improve erectile dysfunction in hemodialysed patients? What is the role of associated factors? *Transplant Proc* 2007;39(4):1029–1032.

7. Rosas SE, Joffe M, Franklin E, et al. Prevalence and determinants of erectile dysfunction in hemodialysis patients. *Kidney Int* 2001;59(6):2259–2266.

8. Laumann EO, Paik A, Rosen RC. Sexual dysfunction in the United States: prevalence and predictors. *JAMA* 1999;281(6):537–544.

9. Handelsman DJ, Dong Q. Hypothalamo-pituitary gonadal axis in chronic renal failure. *Endocrinol Metab Clin North Am* 1993;22(1):145–161.

10. Espinoza R, Gracida C, Cancino J, Ibarra A. Prevalence of erectile dysfunction in kidney transplant recipients. *Transplant Proc* 2006;38(3):916–917.

11. Malavaud B, Rostaing L, Rischmann P, Sarramon JP, Durand D. High prevalence of erectile dysfunction after renal transplantation. *Transplantation* 2000;69(10):2121–2124.

12. Wong JA, Lawen J, Kiberd B, Alkhudair WK. Prevalence and prognostic factors for erectile dysfunction in renal transplant recipients. *Can Urol Assoc J* 2007;1(4):383–387.

13. Rebollo P, Ortega F, Valdes C, et al. Factors associated with erectile dysfunction in male kidney transplant recipients. *Int J Impot Res* 2003;15(6):433–438.

14. Tian Y, Ji ZG, Tang YW, et al. Prevalence and influential factors of erectile dysfunction in male renal transplant recipients: a multiple center survey. *Chin Med J (Engl)* 2008;121(9):795–799.

15. Cummings JM, Boullier JA, Browne BJ, Bose K, Emovon O. Male sexual dysfunction in renal transplant recipients: comparison to men awaiting transplant. *Transplant Proc* 2003;35(2):864–865.

16. Filocamo MT, Zanazzi M, Li Marzi V, et al. Sexual dysfunction in women during dialysis and after renal transplantation. *J Sex Med* 2009;6(11):3125–3131.

17. Nassir A. Sexual function in male patients undergoing treatment for renal failure: a prospective view. *J Sex Med* 2009;6(12):3407–3414.

18. Burra P, De Bona M. Quality of life following organ transplantation. *Transpl Int* 2007;20(5):397–409.

19. Salvatierra O, Jr., Fortmann JL, Belzer FO. Sexual function of males before and after renal transplantation. *Urology* 1975;5(1):64–66.

20. El-Bahnasawy MS, El-Assmy A, El-Sawy E, et al. Critical evaluation of the factors influencing erectile function after renal transplantation. *Int J Impot Res* 2004;16(6):521–526.

21. Shamsa A, Motavalli SM, Aghdam B. Erectile function in end-stage renal disease before and after renal transplantation. *Transplant Proc* 2005;37(7):3087–3089.

22. Peskircioglu L, Tekin MI, Demirag A, Karakayali H, Ozkardes H. Evaluation of erectile function in renal transplant recipients. *Transplant Proc* 1998;30(3):747–749.

23. Burgos FJ, Pascual J, Gomez V, Orofino L, Liano F, Ortuno J. Effect of kidney transplantation and cyclosporine treatment on male sexual performance and hormonal profile: a prospective study. *Transplant Proc* 1997;29(1–2):227–228.

24. El-Bahnasawy MS, El-Assmy A, Dawood A, et al. Effect of the use of internal iliac artery for renal transplantation on penile vascularity and erectile function: a prospective study. *J Urol* 2004;172(6 Pt 1):2335–2339.

25. Tsujimura A, Matsumiya K, Tsuboniwa N, et al. Effect of renal transplantation on sexual function. *Arch Androl* 2002;48(6):467–474.

26. Zhang Y, Guan DL, Ou TW, et al. Sildenafil citrate treatment for erectile dysfunction after kidney transplantation. *Transplant Proc* 2005;37(5):2100–2103.

27. Laupacis A, Keown P, Pus N, et al. A study of the quality of life and cost-utility of renal transplantation. *Kidney Int* 1996;50(1):235–242.

28. Lough ME, Lindsey AM, Shinn JA, Stotts NA. Life satisfaction following heart transplantation. *J Heart Transplant* 1985;4(4):446–449.

29. Mulligan T, Sheehan H, Hanrahan J. Sexual function after heart transplantation. *J Heart Lung Transplant* 1991;10(1 Pt 1):125–128.

30. Phan A, Ishak WW, Shen BJ, et al. Persistent sexual dysfunction impairs quality of life after cardiac transplantation. *J Sex Med* 2010;7(8):2765–2773.

31. Basile A, Maccherini M, Diciolla F, et al. Sexual disorders after heart transplantation. *Transplant Proc* 2001;33(1–2):1917–1919.

32. Tabler JB, Frierson RL. Sexual concerns after heart transplantation. *J Heart Transplant* 1990;9(4):397–403.

33. Wolpowitz A, Barnard CN. Impotence after heart transplantation. *S Afr Med J* 1978;53(18):693.

34. Toda K, Miwa Y, Kuriyama S, et al. Erectile dysfunction in patients with chronic viral liver disease: its relevance to protein malnutrition. *J Gastroenterol* 2005;40(9):894–900.

35. Huyghe E, Kamar N, Wagner F, et al. Erectile dysfunction in end-stage liver disease men. *J Sex Med* 2009;6(5):1395–1401.

36. Sorrell JH, Brown JR. Sexual functioning in patients with end-stage liver disease before and after transplantation. *Liver Transpl* 2006;12(10):1473–1477.

37. Ho JK, Ko HH, Schaeffer DF, et al. Sexual health after orthotopic liver transplantation. *Liver Transpl* 2006;12(10):1478–1484.

38. Hart LK, Milde FK, Zehr PS, Cox DM, Tarara DT, Fearing MO. Survey of sexual concerns among organ transplant recipients. *J Transpl Coord* 1997;7(2):82–87.

39. Bunzel B, Grundbock A, Laczkovics A, Holzinger C, Teufelsbauer H. Quality of life after orthotopic heart transplantation. *J Heart Lung Transplant* 1991;10(3):455–459.

40. Fisher DC, Lake KD, Reutzel TJ, Emery RW. Changes in health-related quality of life and depression in heart transplant recipients. *J Heart Lung Transplant* 1995;14(2):373–381.

41. Grady KL, Jalowiec A, White-Williams C. Improvement in quality of life in patients with heart failure who undergo transplantation. *J Heart Lung Transplant* 1996;15(8):749–757.

42. Mai FM, McKenzie FN, Kostuk WJ. Psychosocial adjustment and quality of life following heart transplantation. *Can J Psychiatry* 1990;35(3):223–227.

43. Harvison A, Jones BM, McBride M, Taylor F, Wright O, Chang VP. Rehabilitation after heart transplantation: the Australian experience. *J Heart Transplant* 1988;7(5):337–341.

44. Rebollo P, Ortega F, Valdes C, et al. Influence of erectile dysfunction on health related quality of life of male kidney transplant patients. *Int J Impot Res* 2004;16(3):282–287.

45. Soffer O. Sexual dysfunction in chronic renal failure. *South Med J* 1980;73(12):1599–1600, 1606.

46. Burra P. Sexual dysfunction after liver transplantation. *Liver Transpl* 2009;15 Suppl 2:S50–56.

47. Samojlik E, Kirschner MA, Ribot S, Szmal E. Changes in the hypothalamic-pituitary-gonadal axis in men after cadaver kidney transplantation and cyclosporine therapy. *J Androl* 1992;13(4):332–336.

48. Fleischer J, McMahon DJ, Hembree W, Addesso V, Longcope C, Shane E. Serum testosterone levels after cardiac transplantation. *Transplantation* 2008;85(6):834–839.

49. Abdel-Hamid IA, Eraky I, Fouda MA, Mansour OE. Role of penile vascular insufficiency in erectile dysfunction in renal transplant recipients. *Int J Impot Res* 2002;14(1):32–37.

50. Pegge NC, Twomey AM, Vaughton K, Gravenor MB, Ramsey MW, Price DE. The role of endothelial dysfunction in the pathophysiology of erectile

dysfunction in diabetes and in determining response to treatment. *Diabet Med* 2006;23(8):873–878.

51. Carrier S, Brock G, Kour NW, Lue TF. Pathophysiology of erectile dysfunction. *Urology* 1993;42(4):468–481.

52. Mark PB, Murphy K, Mohammed AS, Morris ST, Jardine AG. Endothelial dysfunction in renal transplant recipients. *Transplant Proc* 2005;37(9):3805–3807.

53. Hollenberg SM, Klein LW, Parrillo JE, et al. Changes in coronary endothelial function predict progression of allograft vasculopathy after heart transplantation. *J Heart Lung Transplant* 2004;23(3):265–271.

54. Taylor RM. Impotence and the use of the internal iliac artery in renal transplantation: a survey of surgeons' attitudes in the United Kingdom and Ireland. *Transplantation* 1998;65(5):745–746.

55. Nghiem DD, Corry RJ, Picon-Mendez G, Lee HM. Factors influencing male sexual impotence after renal transplantation. *Urology* 1983;21(1):49–52.

56. Feldman HA, Goldstein I, Hatzichristou DG, Krane RJ, McKinlay JB. Impotence and its medical and psychosocial correlates: results of the Massachusetts Male Aging Study. *J Urol* 1994;151(1):54–61.

57. Shabsigh R, Klein LT, Seidman S, Kaplan SA, Lehrhoff BJ, Ritter JS. Increased incidence of depressive symptoms in men with erectile dysfunction. *Urology* 1998;52(5):848–852.

58. Araujo AB, Durante R, Feldman HA, Goldstein I, McKinlay JB. The relationship between depressive symptoms and male erectile dysfunction: cross-sectional results from the Massachusetts Male Aging Study. *Psychosom Med* 1998;60(4):458–465.

59. Seidman SN. Exploring the relationship between depression and erectile dysfunction in aging men. *J Clin Psychiatry* 2002;63 Suppl 5:5–15.

60. Palmer BF. Sexual dysfunction in uremia. *J Am Soc Nephrol* 1999;10(6):1381–1388.

61. Tavallaii SA, Fathi-Ashtiani A, Nasiri M, Assari S, Maleki P, Einollahi B. Correlation between sexual function and postrenal transplant quality of life: does gender matter? *J Sex Med* 2007;4(6):1610–1618.

62. Seethalakshmi L, Flores C, Carboni AA, Bala R, Diamond DA, Menon M. Cyclosporine: its effects on testicular function and fertility in the prepubertal rat. *J Androl* 1990;11(1):17–24.

63. Seethalakshmi L, Flores C, Khauli RB, Diamond DA, Menon M. Evaluation of the effect of experimental cyclosporine toxicity on male reproduction and renal function. Reversal by concomitant human chorionic gonadotropin administration. *Transplantation* 1990;49(1):17–19.

64. Seethalakshmi L, Flores C, Malhotra RK, et al. The mechanism of cyclosporine's action in the inhibition of testosterone biosynthesis by rat Leydig cells in vitro. *Transplantation* 1992;53(1):190–195.

65. Sikka SC, Bhasin S, Coy DC, Koyle MA, Swerdloff RS, Rajfer J. Effects of cyclosporine on the hypothalamic-pituitary-gonadal axis in the male rat: mechanism of action. *Endocrinology* 1988;123(2):1069–1074.

66. Oriji GK, Keiser HR. Role of nitric oxide in cyclosporine A-induced hypertension. *Hypertension* 1998;32(5):849–855.

67. Morris ST, McMurray JJ, Rodger RS, Farmer R, Jardine AG. Endothelial dysfunction in renal transplant recipients maintained on cyclosporine. *Kidney Int* 2000;57(3):1100–1106.

68. Lee J, Kim SW, Kook H, Kang DG, Kim NH, Choi KC. Effects of L-arginine on cyclosporin-induced alterations of vascular NO/cGMP generation. *Nephrol Dial Transplant* 1999;14(11):2634–2638.

69. Esposito C, Fornoni A, Cornacchia F, et al. Cyclosporine induces different responses in human epithelial, endothelial and fibroblast cell cultures. *Kidney Int* 2000;58(1):123–130.

70. Ragazzi E, Meggiato C, Chinellato A, Italiano G, Pagano F, Calabro A. Chronic treatment with cyclosporine A in New Zealand rabbit: aortic and erectile tissue alterations. *Urol Res* 1996;24(6):323–328.

71. Handelsman DJ, McDowell IF, Caterson ID, Tiller DJ, Hall BM, Turtle JR. Testicular function after renal transplantation: comparison of Cyclosporin A with azathioprine and prednisone combination regimes. *Clin Nephrol* 1984;22(3):144–148.

72. Kantarci G, Sahin S, Uras AR, Ergin H. Effects of different calcineurin inhibitors on sex hormone levels in transplanted male patients. *Transplant Proc* 2004;36(1):178–179.

73. Ishikawa A, Ushiyama T, Suzuki K, Fujita K. Serum testosterone levels after renal transplantation. *Transplant Proc* 1996;28(3):1952–1953.

74. Ramirez G, Narvarte J, Bittle PA, Ayers-Chastain C, Dean SE. Cyclosporine-induced alterations in the hypothalamic hypophyseal gonadal axis in transplant patients. *Nephron* 1991;58(1):27–32.

75. Kaufman JM, Hatzichristou DG, Mulhall JP, Fitch WP, Goldstein I. Impotence and chronic renal failure: a study of the hemodynamic pathophysiology. *J Urol* 1994;151(3):612–618.

76. Nickel T, Schlichting CL, Weis M. Drugs modulating endothelial function after transplantation. *Transplantation* 2006;82(1 Suppl):S41–46.

77. Lee S, Coco M, Greenstein SM, Schechner·RS, Tellis VA, Glicklich DG. The effect of sirolimus on sex hormone levels of male renal transplant recipients. *Clin Transplant* 2005;19(2):162–167.

78. Kaczmarek I, Groetzner J, Adamidis I, et al. Sirolimus impairs gonadal function in heart transplant recipients. *Am J Transplant* 2004;4(7):1084–1088.

79. Huyghe E, Zairi A, Nohra J, Kamar N, Plante P, Rostaing L. Gonadal impact of target of rapamycin inhibitors (sirolimus and everolimus) in male patients: an overview. *Transpl Int* 2007;20(4):305–311.

80. Tondolo V, Citterio F, Panocchia N, et al. Gonadal function and immunosuppressive therapy after renal transplantation. *Transplant Proc* 2005;37(4):1915–1917.

81. Rastogi S, Rodriguez JJ, Kapur V, Schwarz ER. Why do patients with heart failure suffer from erectile dysfunction? A critical review and suggestions on how to approach this problem. *Int J Impot Res* 2005;17 Suppl 1:S25–36.

82. Schwarz ER, Rastogi S, Kapur V, Sulemanjee N, Rodriguez JJ. Erectile dysfunction in heart failure patients. *J Am Coll Cardiol* 2006;48(6):1111–1119.

83. Lessan-Pezeshki M, Ghazizadeh S. Sexual and reproductive function in end-stage renal disease and effect of kidney transplantation. *Asian J Androl* 2008;10(3):441–446.

84. Fogari R, Preti P, Derosa G, et al. Effect of antihypertensive treatment with valsartan or atenolol on sexual activity and plasma testosterone in hypertensive men. *Eur J Clin Pharmacol* 2002;58(3):177–180.

85. Fogari R, Zoppi A. Effects of antihypertensive therapy on sexual activity in hypertensive men. *Curr Hypertens Rep* 2002;4(3):202–210.

86. Prieto Castro RM, Anglada Curado FJ, Regueiro Lopez JC, et al. Treatment with sildenafil citrate in renal transplant patients with erectile dysfunction. *BJU Int* 2001;88(3):241–243.

87. Lasaponara F, Paradiso M, Milan MG, et al. Erectile dysfunction after kidney transplantation: our 22 years of experience. *Transplant Proc* 2004;36(3):502–504.

88. Barry JM. Treating erectile dysfunction in renal transplant recipients. *Drugs* 2007;67(7):975–983.

89. Chatterjee R, Wood S, McGarrigle HH, Lees WR, Ralph DJ, Neild GH. A novel therapy with testosterone and sildenafil for erectile dysfunction in patients on renal dialysis or after renal transplantation. *J Fam Plann Reprod Health Care* 2004;30(2):88–90.

90. Sharma RK, Prasad N, Gupta A, Kapoor R. Treatment of erectile dysfunction with sildenafil citrate in renal allograft recipients: a randomized, double-blind, placebo-controlled, crossover trial. *Am J Kidney Dis* 2006;48(1):128–133.

91. Barrou B, Cuzin B, Malavaud B, et al. Early experience with sildenafil for the treatment of erectile dysfunction in renal transplant recipients. *Nephrol Dial Transplant* 2003;18(2):411–417.

92. Christ B, Brockmeier D, Hauck EW, Kamali-Ernst S. Investigation on interaction between tacrolimus and sildenafil in kidney-transplanted patients with erectile dysfunction. *Int J Clin Pharmacol Ther* 2004;42(3):149–156.

93. Christ B, Brockmeier D, Hauck EW, Friemann S. Interactions of sildenafil and tacrolimus in men with erectile dysfunction after kidney transplantation. *Urology* 2001;58(4):589–593.

94. Espinoza R, Melchor JL, Gracida C. Sildenafil (Viagra) in kidney transplant recipients with erectile dysfunction. *Transplant Proc* 2002;34(1):408–409.

95. Malavaud B, Rostaing L, Tran-Van T, Tack I, Ader JL. Transient renal effects of sildenafil in male kidney transplant recipients. *Transplantation* 2001;72(7):1331–1333.

96. Schofield RS, Edwards DG, Schuler BT, et al. Vascular effects of sildenafil in hypertensive cardiac transplant recipients. *Am J Hypertens* 2003;16(10):874–877.

97. Wren FJ, Jarowenko MV, Burg J, Boehmer J. Incidence of erectile dysfunction and efficacy of sildenafil in the cardiac transplantation patient. *J Heart Lung Transplant* 2001;20(2):246.

98. Demir E, Balal M, Paydas S, Sertdemir Y, Erken U. Efficacy and safety of vardenafil in renal transplant recipients with erectile dysfunction. *Transplant Proc* 2006;38(5):1379–1381.

99. Mansi MK, Alkhudair WK, Huraib S. Treatment of erectile dysfunction after kidney transplantation with intracavernosal self-injection of prostaglandin E1. *J Urol* 1998;159(6):1927–1930.

100. Livi U, Faggian G, Sorbara C, et al. Use of prostaglandin E1 in the treatment of sexual impotence after heart transplantation: initial clinical experience. *J Heart Lung Transplant* 1993;12(3):484–486.

101. Sidi AA, Peng W, Sanseau C, Lange PH. Penile prosthesis surgery in the treatment of impotence in the immunosuppressed man. *J Urol* 1987;137(4):681–682.

102. Kabalin JN, Kessler R. Successful implantation of penile prostheses in organ transplant patients. *Urology* 1989;33(4):282–284.

103. Rowe SJ, Montague DK, Steinmuller DR, Lakin MM, Novick AC. Treatment of organic impotence with penile prosthesis in renal transplant patients. *Urology* 1993;41(1):16–20.

104. Walther PJ, Andriani RT, Maggio MI, Carson CC, 3rd. Fournier's gangrene: a complication of penile prosthetic implantation in a renal transplant patient. *J Urol* 1987;137(2):299–300.

105. Cuellar DC, Sklar GN. Penile prosthesis in the organ transplant recipient. *Urology* 2001;57(1):138–141.

Chapter 10

Living with Erectile Dysfunction, the Man's and the Partner's Perspective, and Prevention of Erectile Dysfunction

Paul D. Thompson and Ernst R. Schwarz

Introduction

Erectile dysfunction (ED) is a common condition, experienced by up to 22% of men in the United States and projected to affect 322 million worldwide by the year 2025 (1). The incidence of ED increases with age, similar to the increase of other age-related diseases (coronary artery disease, hypertension, diabetes). The Massachusetts Male Aging Study (2) revealed that the incidence of complete impotence tripled from 5% at 40 years to 15% at 70 years. ED has an equal effect on both partners in a relationship and has been implicated as the primary cause of divorce in 20% of failed marriages. The man may experience guilt or embarrassment and begin to withdraw from the relationship. ED has been noted to be associated with serious self-esteem problems, leading to the demise of a large percentage of affected relationships (3). This withdrawal from the relationship may lead to the partner questioning her attractiveness and subsequently lowering her self-esteem. This ultimately leads to humiliation, frustration, and a mutual withdrawal from the relationship.

Even with multiple treatment options available, not all men will seek treatment. Many require support from their partner to admit the fact that there is a problem. The best alternative is to avoid ED at all costs. This can be done in a proactive manner through lifestyle changes, including diet, exercise, and avoidance of certain substances.

ED: The Man's Perspective

There is much written about the devastating effects of ED on the male psyche. These feelings range from low self-esteem to pure hopelessness. These feelings often are associated with increasing episodes of ED, leading to a vicious cycle of ED and depression. It has been reported that 100% of men with some form of ED also suffer a decrease in self-esteem, with subsequent friction in their relationship. The level of damage to self-image is highly influenced by the man's avocation or occupation (4). The MALES Phase I study (5), with over 27,000 participants from eight countries, showed that not all stereotypes associated with ED hold true for all men. Men with qualities like honor, self-reliance, and respect from friends defined masculinity as more than an erection and a sexual act. This went against many of the previously held concepts regarding men with ED, and it extended across all nationalities and ages. This supports the theory that the degree of negative effect from ED is directly influenced by the individual's prior emotional health.

Further influences on quality of life are age and degree of severity. Younger men have more pronounced worries than their older counterparts; older men regardless of the degree of ED have a higher overall sexual satisfaction, even in the face of lower sexual desire. In younger men the degree of ED has a much greater influence on sexual satisfaction compared to their older counterparts (6). Men with ED have been noted to have lower satisfaction not only with their sex life but also with their life in general. Interestingly, these same men with ED, when compared to controls, had higher satisfaction scores regarding their financial status and their leisure time activities (7). When comparing individuals with moderate and severe ED, there were no significant differences regarding their overall life satisfaction.

ED: The Partner's Perspective

Research has demonstrated that a decline in sexual activity occurs in both men and women as they age. The reasons are very different: for men, it is due to health, medications, and age. In women it is more likely due to loss of a functional partner; their health is less of a factor (8). When treatment is sought, in the majority of cases the partner is left out of the treatment equation by both the physician and the man.

Research has indicated that ED and its treatment are best handled as a couple's problem, and the treatment affects both the man and the partner equally. Treatment can lead to the partner experiencing the perception of improved emotional closeness, improved communication, and a feeling that the relationship is more stable and loving (9). The average man with ED presents to his primary care physician alone. Questions regarding lack of partner accompaniment indicated that the spouse was previously committed (58%), he didn't think of it (24%), and he didn't know it was possible (15%) (10). This indicates that communication with the patient prior to the visit is helpful and leads to a more productive consultation and satisfied couple. When questioned regarding their partner's response to ED, the results revealed disappointment (29%), vexation (27%), frustration (17%) and finally acceptance, but most commonly understanding (77%) (10). In view of the above, it is essential to include the partner in the treatment from the outset to obtain the best outcome. Even in the face of the above, it has been shown that 44% of the partners remained satisfied with their sexual relationship and 54% with their sex life.

The partner's perception of the nature and cause of ED is associated with the man's willingness to seek treatment and his openness to using said treatment. The partner's satisfaction with the relationship prior to ED, her perception of ED and its effect on quality of life, her openness to treatment options, and her willingness to deal with treatment have a very significant influence on the man seeking treatment (11). This response by the partner was reported in other studies as well. For some partners there was a sense of frustration and hopelessness, but for many it stimulated them to increase nonphysical intimacy and communication regarding sex (12). This demonstrates the importance of the couple's relationship and their ability to communicate prior to the development of ED.

Impact of Treatment

Once medical intervention is sought, it is important to the success of the treatment that the partner be included from the outset and that counseling includes information regarding the incidence of ED as well as the many treatment options available. The introduction to treatment and cause can be shared with the couple before they present for the initial consultation. When done in this manner, the partner has adequate time to digest the information and formulate questions pertinent to the cause and treatment options. This improves the acceptance of ED by the partner, alleviating any guilt or blame she may feel, making her more understanding and compassionate to her partner. Providing literature before the initial clinic visit does require a preconsultation interview, but it pays off with increased patient satisfaction and compliance (13).

Prior to treatment, the partners of patients with ED engage in sexual activity less frequently than prior to the development of ED. The majority do not experience sexual desire, arousal, or orgasm, and most were not satisfied with their sexual relationship after ED. When this group received treatment, the incidence of sexual desire, arousal, and orgasm in the partner was markedly increased. ED has a significant effect on the partner's sexual experience; treatment can significantly reverse this phenomenon, leading to a more satisfying sexual relationship for both partners (14).

Prevention of ED

In most cases ED is a preventable disease, but prevention requires that individuals be educated and informed about risk factors. Well-educated and informed individuals can prevent and/or delay the onset of debilitating diseases that many associate with the aging process. When questioned about risk factors associated with ED, greater than 50% of individuals can't name a single one. The most common source of information comes from the Internet and primary care physicians. Individuals using the Internet are better informed, younger, and better educated (15). Since the risk factors for ED are the same as for many other serious diseases, there is a great need to educate the population regarding them.

Risk factors associated with ED are strikingly similar to those of cardiovascular disease. Obesity, metabolic syndrome, hypertension, inactivity, diabetes, and smoking are all positively associated with ED and cardiovascular disease. Exercise and weight control secondary to a healthier diet are inversely associated with ED and cardiovascular disease. These habits not only decrease the incidence of both ED and cardiovascular disease but also decrease inflammation and subsequently improve endothelial health. Knowing that these risk factors are associated with ED may be a motivating factor to convince men to adopt a healthier life style (16–19).

Smoking

Smoking prevalence in the United States has declined in the past 40-plus years but has stalled in the past 5 to 10 years. According to the Centers for Disease Control and Prevention, the rate in 1965 was 42% and as of 2009 that rate for adults (18 years and older) was 20.6% (23.5% male and 17.5% female, with education level being inversely proportional to smoking rate). There is an increased incidence of ED in individuals who smoked at any time. The association appears to be dose-dependent and greatest in those who continue to smoke (20).

A study in the *European Journal of Urology* found an association with smoking and demonstrated that it was dose-dependent. Men with a 20 pack-year history of smoking had a statistically significant increase in the incidence of ED. Nonsmokers who were exposed to secondhand smoke had a moderately increased risk of ED (21). This information confirms what we have thought for some time: smoking is a risk factor not only for cardiovascular disease but also for ED. The mechanism of action has not been definitively demonstrated, but it would appear to be inflammatory in nature with subsequent endothelial damage.

Lifestyle and Nutrition

There are several risk factors that when modified can greatly decrease the incidence and/or progression of ED, including obesity, sedentary lifestyle, smoking, and alcohol consumption. The timing of these modifications also has an effect on ED: midlife changes including a decrease in alcohol consumption, cessation of smoking, and weight loss appeared to have little effect on ED, while an increase in physical activity reduced the incidence of ED, even when initiated late in life. A study from the New England Research Institute found that adopting a healthy lifestyle early in one's life was the best approach to preventing or decreasing the incidence of ED in later life (22). One further lifestyle change often not considered is the relationship between the frequency of sexual intercourse and the development of ED: men who had sexual intercourse less than once a week had twice the incidence of ED compared to men who had sexual intercourse once a week or more (23). The conclusion from this study was that regular intercourse protected men from ED and that it also had an impact on their overall health and quality of life. The lifestyle changes mentioned above will be reviewed in detail later in the chapter. These lifestyle changes result in a decrease in inflammation, resulting in improved endothelial health. This results in improved vascular blood flow and is beneficial in reducing ED and coronary artery disease (24).

Nutrients and Botanicals (Supplements)

Currently there is an abundance of over-the-counter supplements, plant products, and home remedies claiming to be the "natural" answer to ED. While it is possible that some of these products may be of benefit to ED patients, there is very limited research, if any, demonstrating said benefits. The placebo effect may play the largest role in many of the supplements' success. The placebo effect has been demonstrated to be as high as 25% to 50% in some trials. Supplements enjoying this placebo effect can be very financially successful, stimulating other formulations to enter the market with hopes of similar outcomes (25).

Our role as clinicians is to be familiar with these supplements and to be able to explain the placebo effect. Even so, the patient may continue to use the supplement if he experiences erectile improvement. There need to be more randomized trials of these supplements if they are going to be considered mainstream, and there should be a control mechanism for manufacturing and labeling of these supplements.

Mental Health and Depression

There is an established association between depression and ED; in fact, it becomes difficult to distinguish whether the depression caused the ED or the ED caused the depression. In the majority of patients with severe depression, when they are successfully treated the ED resolves. In patients with minor depression, when their ED is corrected their mood in the majority of cases is improved. This demonstrates the importance of clinicians being able to diagnose not only ED but also depression. Patients receiving treatment for ED who have untreated mild to moderate depression often stop their treatment for their ED. This may lead to worsening depression, which may become life threatening (26). This demonstrates the need to treat the entire patient and not focus on one diagnosis. This is done by performing a thorough history and physical and discussing with the patient his feeling about his current situation.

Obesity

Obesity increases a man's risk of ED by 30% to 90% over that of leaner men. The high incidence of ED in men with cardiovascular disease suggests that there is a vascular component to ED in these individuals. Men with ED have an increased incidence of metabolic syndrome, hypertension, and insulin resistance. Of men who adopt a healthy lifestyle, increase their physical activity, and lose weight, one third will regain their sexual function after 2 years. Evidence suggests that by adopting a healthier lifestyle (Mediterranean-like diet with an increase in physical activity), individuals can prevent cardiovascular disease, ED, and premature death. Studies have revealed that an obese 40-year-old man has a 7-year decrease in life expectancy. The lifestyle changes lead to an improvement of metabolic disturbances with a decrease in inflammatory markers and improved endothelial health, resulting in an increased life expectancy. With the current epidemic proportions of obesity, physicians must be fluent discussing metabolic abnormalities and their remedies. If we are to reverse the obesity epidemic, we must be more knowledgeable about nutrition and exercise plans. Society spends a disproportionate amount of its health care dollars on obesity and associated diseases. Adopting a healthy lifestyle will improve society's overall health, decreasing the incidence of cardiovascular disease, diabetes, hypertension, and ED. At the same time this will relieve the large burden on our overextended medical system, resulting in lower health care costs and improved quality of life for all (24, 27, 28).

Exercise

There are numerous studies examining the benefits of healthy lifestyles on ED. A healthy lifestyle includes moderate to no alcohol consumption, a Mediterranean-like diet, no smoking, and physical activity (exercise). Studies have shown that individuals who adopt these healthy habits have a decreased incidence of ED as well as cardiovascular disease, diabetes, hypertension, and obesity. The timing of initiation of this healthy lifestyle plays a role in ED as well. Those waiting until midlife to change their diet, quit smoking, and decrease alcohol consumption often see very little improvement of their ED and the impending development of ED. Exercise, on the other hand, appears to benefit the individual even when initiated in midlife, with a reduction in ED both immediately and in later years (17, 18, 22).

The exercise need not be as structured as many think. There are significant benefits to simply being less sedentary. Walks, yard work, or participating in an organized beginner exercise class may be enough to secure significant benefits in terms of weight reduction, drop in blood pressure, and better glucose control. These changes have an effect on inflammation and endothelial health, leading to a decrease in all vascular diseases, including ED and cardiovascular disease (18).

Hormonal Optimization

Testosterone is required for erectile function; it has been shown that in hypogonadal men testosterone replacement restores both libido and erectile function (29). With this increase in testosterone there is an associated increase in free testosterone, which has a direct effect on erectile function and libido (30). There has been conclusive evidence of a direct link with hormones and erectile function (31). The controversy comes in defining normal and optimal testosterone levels. There is a considerable difference between optimal and normal levels; most labs report the normal range extends from 250 to 900. More important is the free testosterone level. When levels are optimal we see a decrease in cardiovascular disease, hypertension, diabetes, and ED. Associated with these changes are increases in lean muscle mass (32), bone mineral density (33), feeling of well-being (34), and erectile function (29).

Conclusion

ED is a common problem that affects both partners in a relationship equally and often leads to the demise of that relationship. Treatment is much more successful when both partners participate and are present at the initial evaluation and at ongoing visits with the physician. The treatment options require that the patient make lifestyle changes that will require the support of his partner. Individuals can decrease the incidence of this disease by making some minor changes in their lifestyle; these changes will at the same time improve their overall health and quality of life.

References

1. Seftel AD. *Male and Female Sexual Dysfunction*. Mosby: 2004.

2. Feldman HA, et al. Impotence and its medical and psychosocial correlates: results of the Massachusetts Male Aging Study. *J Urol* 1994;1:54.

3. Tomlinson J, Wright D. Impact of erectile dysfunction and its subsequent treatment with sildenafil. *BMJ* 2004;328.

4. Kingsberg SA. The psychological impact of aging on sexuality and relationships. *J Womens Health Gender Based Med* 2000;9(Suppl 1):S33–38.

5. Sand MS, Fisher W, Rosen R, Heiman J, Eardley I. Erectile dysfunction and constructs of masculinity and quality of life in the multinational Men's Attitudes to Life events and Sexuality (MALES) study. *J Sex Med* 2008;5(3):583–594.

6. Gralla O, Knoll N, et al. Worry, desire and sexual satisfaction and their association with severity of ED and age. *J Sex Med* 2008;5(11):2645–2655.

7. Mallis D, Moisidis K, et al. Moderate and severe erectile dysfunction equally affects life satisfaction. *J Sex Med* 2006;3(3):442–449.

8. Avis NE. Sexual function and aging in men and women. *J Gend Specif Med* 200;3(2):37–41.

9. McCabe MP, O'Connor EJ, Conaglen JV, Conaglen HM. Impact of oral ED medication on female partners' relationship satisfaction. *J Sex Med* 2011;8(2):479–483.

10. Delavierre D, Poisson E. Female partners confronted with erectile dysfunction. A series of 137 patients. *Prog Urol* 2011;21(1):59–66.

11. Fisher WA, Eardley I, McCabe M, Sand M. Erectile dysfunction is a shared sexual concern of couples. *J Sex Med* 2009;(11):3111–3124.

12. O'Connor E, McCabe M, Conaglen H, Conaglen J. Attitudes and experiences: Qualitative perspectives on erectile dysfunction from the female partner. *J Health Psychol* 2012;17(1):3–13.

13. Berner MM, Leiber C, Kriston L, Stodden V, Gunzler C. Effects of written information material on help-seeking behavior in patients with erectile dysfunction. *J Sex Med* 2008;5(2):436–447.

14. Fisher WA, Rosen RC, Eardley I, Sand M, Goldstein I. Sexual experience of female partners of men with erectile dysfunction. *J Sex Med* 2005;2(5):675–684.

15. Baumgartner MK, Hermanns T, Cohen A, Schid DM, Seifert B, Sulserl T, Strebel RT. Patients' knowledge about risk factors for erectile dysfunction is poor. *J Sex Med* 2008;5(10):2399–2404.

16. Selvin E, Burnett AL, Platz EA. Prevalence and risk factors for erectile dysfunction in the U.S. *Am J Med* 2007;120(2):151–157.

17. Bacon CG, Mittleman MA, Kawachi I, Giovannucci E, Glasser DB, Rimm EB. A prospective study of risk factors for erectile dysfunction. *J Urol* 2006;176(1):217–221.

18. Jackson G. The importance of risk factor reduction in erectile dysfunction. *Curr Urol Rep* 2007;8(6):463–466.

19. Pommerville P. Erectile dysfunction: an overview. *Can J Urol* 2003(Suppl 1):2–6.

20. Gades NM, Nehra A, Jacobson DJ, McGree ME, Girman CJ, Rhodes T, Roberts RO, Lieber MM, Jacobson SJ. Association between smoking and erectile dysfunction: A population-based study. *Am J Epidemiol* 2005;161(4):346–351.

21. Kupelian V, Link CL, Mckinlay JB. Association between smoking, passive smoking and erectile dysfunction: Results from the Boston Area Community Health (BACH) survey. *Eur Urol* 2007;52(2):416–422.

22. Derby C, Mohr B, Goldstein I, Feldman HA, Johannes CB, McKinlay J. Modifiable risk factors and erectile dysfunction: Can lifestyle changes modify risks? *Urology* 56(2):302–306.

23. Koskmaki J, Shiri R, Tammela T, Hakkinen J, Hakama M Auvinen A. Regular intercourse protects against erectile dysfunction: Tampere Aging Male Urologic Study. *Am J Med* 2008;121(7):592–596.

24. Jackson G. The importance of risk factor reduction in erectile dysfunction. *Curr Urol Rep* 2007;8(6):463–466.

25. Moyad MA. Dietary supplements and other alternative medicines for erectile dysfunction. What do I tell my patients? *Urol Clin North Am* 2002;29(1):11–22.

26. Seagraves RT. Depression and erectile dysfunction. *Postgrad Med* 2000;107(suppl Educational):24–27.

27. Esposito K, Giugliano D. Obesity, the metabolic syndrome and sexual dysfunction. *Int J Impot Res* 2005;175:391–398.

28. Esposito K, Giugliano F, Ciotola M, De Sio M, D'Armiento M, Giugliano D. Obesity and sexual dysfunction, male and female. *Int J Impot Res* 2008;20(4):358–365.

29. Bancroft J, Wu FC. Changes in erectile responsiveness during androgen replacement therapy. *Arch Sex Behav* 1983;12:59–66.

30. Guay AT, Jacobson J Perez J, Hodge MB, Velaquez E. Clomiphene increases free testosterone levels in men with both secondary hypogonadism and erectile dysfunction. *Int J Impot Res* 2003;15(3):156–165.

31. Goldstein I. Relation of sex steroid hormones to genital tissue structure and arousal. *Int J Impot Res* 2003;15:389–390.

32. Tenover JS. Male hormonal changes with aging. In: *Endocrinology and Metabolism in the Elderly*. Blackwell Scientific; 1992:243–261.

33. Jackson JA, Kleerekoper M, Parfitt AM, et al. Bone histomorphometry in hypogonadal and eugonadal men with spinal osteoporosis. *J Clin Endocrinol Metab* 1987;65(1):53–58.

34. Marin P, Holmang S, Gustafsson E, et al. Androgen treatment of abdominally obese men. *Obesity Res* 1993;1:245–251.

Chapter 11

Ongoing and Future Research

Anthony J. Bella and Rany Shamloul

Introduction

Advances in the understanding of the physiological mechanisms responsible for penile erection and pathophysiologies resulting in erectile dysfunction (ED) have led to the development of novel treatments such as the oral phosphodiesterase-5 (PDE-5) inhibitor class of agents, which can, in the majority of cases, successfully treat ED. However, our knowledge of the underlying biological events that govern the erectile response remains incomplete; as new molecular targets or mechanisms are identified, the potential exists for refining or redefining treatments for compromised erectile function. This chapter examines ongoing research and provides a look into the "translational" future of patient management, including such exciting opportunities for personalized and target-specific intervention as gene and growth factor therapy, stem cell and cell-based therapies, and regenerative medicine.

Translational Molecular Signaling Targets

NO and the Guanylate Cyclase/cGMP Pathway

Nitric oxide (NO), a gaseous neurotransmitter, plays a primary role in the relaxation of the corpora cavernosa smooth muscle and vasculature (1–4). Neuronal (nNOS) and endothelial (eNOS) nitric oxide synthase of the corpora cavernosa may be the source of NO (5–7). In addition to second-messenger cGMP transduction of the signal, complementary molecular targets resulting in the relaxation of penile smooth muscle remain incompletely elucidated. Two different cGMP-dependent protein kinases (cGK I and II) have been identified in mammals. Inactivation of cGKI in mice abolishes both NO/cGMP-dependent relaxation of vascular and intestinal smooth muscle and the inhibition of platelet aggregation, causing hypertension, intestinal dysmotility, and abnormal hemostasis (8). Sadeghipour and colleagues (9) suggested that lithium, by interfering with the NO pathway in both endothelium and nitrergic nerve, can result in impairment of both the endothelium and nonadrenergic, noncholinergic-mediated relaxation of rat corpora cavernosa. Analysis of the NO/cGMP-induced relaxation clearly shows that cGKI is the major mediator of the cGMP signaling cascade in murine corpora cavernosa tissue. Its absence cannot be compensated for by the cAMP signaling cascade (10). Thus, it appears from these findings that cGKI may be an important player in the signal cascade leading to penile erection (11).

The expression of cGMP-dependent protein kinase (PKG)1α and PKG1β in the corpora cavernosa and the effect of adenoviral gene transfer of PKG1α to the erectile compartment in a rat model of diabetes has been recently studied (12). PKG1α and PKG1β activities were found to be reduced in the erectile tissue of the diabetic rat, while gene transfer of PKG1α to the penis restored PKG activity and erectile function. The authors concluded that gene therapy procedures targeting PKG1α might be a promising therapeutic approach to overcome diabetic ED resistant to oral pharmacotherapy.

Angulo and colleagues evaluated the influence of protein kinase C (PKC) activity on penile smooth muscle tone in tissues from diabetic and nondiabetic men with ED, reporting that overactivity of PKC in diabetes mellitus may be responsible for enhanced contraction and reduced endothelium-dependent relaxation of human corpora cavernosa smooth muscle and could ultimately result in ED (13).

Modulating other gaseous neurotransmitters may eventually modulate steps of the erectile process or counter pathological deficiencies. For example, significant, positive experimental effects of the heme oxygenase/carbon monoxide (HO/CO) system have been identified, yet the data are still in their infancy and the clinical relevance remains undetermined (14).

The RhoA/Rho-kinase Pathway

A major mechanism of the calcium sensitization of smooth muscle contraction is through the inhibition of the smooth muscle myosin light chain phosphatase (Fig. 11.1). Several studies have revealed important roles for the small GTPase RhoA and its effector, Rho-associated kinase (Rho-kinase), in calcium-independent regulation of smooth muscle contraction; this area of research is noteworthy for its promise. The RhoA/Rhokinase pathway modulates the level of phosphorylation of the myosin light chain of myosin II, mainly through inhibition of myosin phosphatase (15, 16). This calcium-sensitizing RhoA/Rhokinase pathway may also play a synergistic role in cavernosal vasoconstriction to maintain penile flaccidity (17). Rho-kinase is known to inhibit myosin light chain phosphatase and to directly phosphorylate myosin light chains, altogether resulting in a net increase in activated myosin and the promotion of cellular contraction (11). Although Rho-kinase protein and mRNA have been detected in corpora cavernosa tissue, the role of Rho-kinase in the regulation of corpora cavernosa tone is not established. Jin and Burnett (18) examined the role of Rho-kinase in corpora cavernosa tone and found that Rho-kinase antagonism stimulated rat penile erection independently of NO and suggested that this principle could be a potential alternate avenue for the treatment of ED.

Another study (19) investigated the effect of testosterone on RhoA/Rho-kinase signaling in diabetes and found that overexpression of RhoA/Rho-kinase signaling contributes to diabetes-related ED. One of the proposed mechanisms responsible for diabetes-related ED is overactivity of RhoA/Rho-kinase signaling, as seen in experimental models of diabetes. Gao and colleagues (20) suggested that impaired erectile function with aging in Sprague-Dawley rats is associated with the imbalance between nNOS and Rho-kinase activity and that the Rho-kinase inhibitor, Y-27632, could improve erectile function in aged Sprague-Dawley

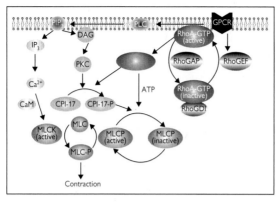

Figure 11.1 Ca^{2+} sensitization and Ca^{2+}-dependent pathways in penile smooth muscle. Stimulation of GPCRs leads to the activation of both Ca^{2+} sensitization and Ca^{2+}-dependent pathways. PLC catalyses PIP2 into IP3 and DAG. IP3 increases intracellular Ca^{2+} levels and, together with CaM (calmodulin), Ca^{2+} activates MLCK. MLCK then phosphorylates MLC, resulting in smooth muscle contraction. After activation by DAG, PKC phosphorylates CPI-17. Phosphorylated CPI-17 has a high affinity for the catalytic subunit of MLCP and decreases MLCP activity through phosphorylation. Activation of GPCRs also stimulates RhoGEF activity, which facilitates the exchange of GTP for GDP on RhoA and dissociates RhoA from RhoGDI. The active RhoA-GTP translocates from the cytosol to the plasma membrane and activates Rho-kinase. Subsequently, Rho-kinase phosphorylates the targeting subunit of MLCP, leading to increased MLC phosphorylation. In addition, Rho-kinase has been shown to phosphorylate CPI-17. Meanwhile, RhoGAP accelerates the intrinsic GTPase activity of RhoA and promotes hydrolysis of GTP; thus, inactive RhoA-GDP re-associates with RhoGDI and relocates to the cytosol.[18]

rats by adjusting this imbalance. Theoretically, suppression of an increased RhoA/Rho-kinase activity is an attractive therapeutic principle in ED. However, the ubiquitous occurrence of the Rho/Rho-kinase pathway limits the use of Rho-kinase inhibitors. If regulators of RhoA/Rho-kinase exclusively expressed in penile tissue can be illustrated, then they can be considered a potential treatment of ED (11).

Centrally Acting Agents

Dopamine agonists, including apomorphine, potentiate penile erection by activation of D2 (21). Recent research demonstrated that D2 receptors may be divided into D2 (long and short variants), D3, and D4 receptor subtypes (22). Interestingly, selective D4 agonists or partial agonists induce penile erection when injected systemically or into the paraventricular nucleus of the hypothalamus (23). These promising studies make central D4 receptors important potential targets for the development of drugs that can successfully treat ED.

Endothelins

Endothelins have been demonstrated in penile erectile tissues and may contribute to the maintenance of corpora cavernosa smooth muscle tone (24–26).

In the endothelium of human corpora cavernosa tissue, intense endothelin-like immunoreactivity has been observed and binding sites for endothelin 1 (ET 1) have been demonstrated by autoradiography in the vessels and in corpora cavernosa tissue (27).

ET-1 potently induces slowly developing, long-lasting contractions in different smooth muscles of the penis: the corpora cavernosa, cavernous artery, deep dorsal vein, and penile circumflex veins. Contractions can also be evoked in human corpora cavernosa tissue by ET-2 and ET-3, although these peptides have a lower potency than ET-1 (28, 29). In a rat model of chronic cocaine administration, Kendirci and colleagues (30) found significantly increased plasma levels of big-ET-1 in the cocaine treatment group compared with control animals. In the penis, cocaine administration significantly increased ETA receptor expression compared with saline controls, while ETB receptor expression was not altered. Cocaine-treated rats also showed significantly decreased endothelial NOS (eNOS) expression and NO production. The authors concluded that cocaine administration significantly reduces erectile function in rats and that the pathophysiological mechanisms likely involved include increased plasma levels of big-ET-1, increased penile ETA receptor expression, and reduced penile eNOS expression.

Clinical research reported conflicting results on the role of ET-1 in penile detumescence. Becker and colleagues (31) reported that in healthy males, no changes in ET-1 or ET-2 levels were observed in the systemic and cavernosal blood during penile tumescence, rigidity, and detumescence, while higher levels were found in patients with ED in the systemic circulation than in the cavernosal blood during penile flaccidity and detumescence. However, they concluded that their data did not support speculations regarding the involvement of ET-1 in the pathophysiology of ED. On the other hand, El Melegy and colleagues (32) found significantly greater mean plasma levels of ET-1 in the venous blood of patients with ED than in controls, suggesting that ET-1 could be a clinical marker of diffuse endothelial disease manifested by ED. So far, the only published pilot clinical study with selective ETA receptor antagonists failed to show enhancement of erectile responses in men with mild to moderate ED (33).

Growth Factor and Cytokine Targets for ED

Optimizing growth factor response or growth factors as therapeutics represents another potential strategy for the treatment of ED (34). This therapy utilizes neuroprotective and vasculoprotective interventions targeting specific biological mechanisms involved in the erectile response that are damaged either by neuropathic disease or injury.

One of the major fields for the application of growth factor therapy in ED, neuromodulation, grew out of the interest in preserving erectile function in men undergoing treatments for prostate cancer and other pelvic malignancies in which ED regularly occurs as a consequence of surgically traumatized cavernous nerves (35, 36). Neurotrophic molecules of particular interest include both classic neurotrophins as well as atypical neurotrophic factors. In experimental rat models of cavernous nerve grafting, nerve growth factor (NGF) and acidic fibroblast growth factor (FGF) enhanced nerve function recovery in the penis and facilitated electrophysiologically induced erectile responses (37, 38). Recent studies have pointed to the important role of the JAK/STAT signaling pathway in mediating the effects of brain-derived neurotrophic factor-induced functional recovery (39–41). The discovery of immunophilins in nerve tissue that operate as specialized receptors for neuroprotection and neuroregeneration has led to their being investigated as a basis for therapy for conditions ranging from neurodegenerative disorders to peripheral nerve injury (42, 43).

Another important growth factor treatment strategy that has shown early promising results in preclinical studies is the cytokine hormone erythropoietin. Erythropoietin, known to have impressive neurotrophic effects for penile nerve function preservation, as demonstrated in animal models of cavernous nerve injury, has also shown potential benefit in men undergoing radical prostatectomy who were involved in a small, nonblinded clinical trial (44, 45).

Another subgroup of growth factor study is the potential application of angiogenic and vascular cytokines to promote erectile function. For example, vascular endothelial growth factor (VEGF), a direct-acting specific endothelial cell mitogen and angiogenic factor, has been most significantly studied in relationship to genital vasculature. In animal models of vasculogenic ED, intracavernous delivery of VEGF effectively restored erectile function (46, 47). Mechanisms involved in these very exciting effects include increasing endothelial cell content (48) and causing both eNOS upregulation (49) and direct activation by Akt phosphorylation in the corpora cavernosa (50).

Finally, a number of researchers explored the value of modulation of pro-inflammatory cytokines, well-described mediators of endothelial dysfunction, to improve erectile function. Levels of tumor necrosis factor-alpha (TNF-α), a well-known pro-inflammatory cytokine involved in multiple cardiovascular diseases, were found to be elevated in men with ED. Carneiro and colleagues studied erection responses and molecular mechanisms operating at the penile level in genetically TNF-α knockout mice (51). Surprisingly, these mice demonstrated improved erections *in vivo* and *in vitro* (i.e., increased NO-dependent cavernosal tissue relaxation and diminished sympathetically mediated effects) in association with increased protein expressions of both neuronal and eNOS enzymes in cavernosal tissue compared with control animals (51). Thus, it is acceptable to state that the suppression of eNOS expression by TNF-α constitutes a mechanism for its pro-erectile effect. Taken together, these data suggest that anti-TNF-α therapies may be effective in treating forms of ED associated with endothelial dysfunction (11).

Gene Therapy

Gene therapy to treat inherited and acquired diseases represents a paradigm shift forward in medicine, although at this stage it truly remains a future therapy in the context of erectile restoration. The concept of gene transfer is to introduce into specific somatic cells new genetic material that will produce a beneficial effect by replacing or correcting a defective or deficient gene in the nucleus of the cell (52). This approach has the advantage that the introduced gene will produce a specific protein product with a specific action in the cell. This is in contrast to drug-based therapies, which may produce multiple effects in nonspecific cell and organ groups (53, 54). More recently, gene therapy has been employed for the treatment of a wide range of disorders, including ED. Since the first preclinical publications of the value of gene therapy for ED treatment, numerous research teams have confirmed the viability of this treatment modality, and numerous strategies have been employed to date.

Because ED generally precedes or presents simultaneously with cardiovascular risk factors, and furthermore because cardiovascular disease has been clearly associated with endothelial dysfunction, it is logical to conclude that ED often results from endothelial dysfunction of the penile vasculature (11, 54). As a result, several gene therapy strategies have been employed to manipulate this cell and enhance the effects generated to treat the disease condition, and many of these studies have been recently reviewed (54). The main focus of all these strategies was the modulation of expression of NOS isoforms, SOD, and most recently HO-1. In all cases the goal is the same: to increase cGMP levels/ NO bioavailability.

The vascular factor is an important determinant of overall erectile function, and thus it is feasible to use angiogenesis to increase the vascularity of the penis and provide an increased blood flow component to the erectile process. Currently, VEGF gene transfer techniques are being applied to the treatment of other ischemic cardiovascular diseases such as myocardial ischemia (55). The direct intracorporal injection of VEGF in a rat model of vascular insufficiency had restorative effects on the nerve-stimulated intracavernous pressure response (56–59) and thus provided "proof of concept" for this approach (47). Dr. Lue and colleagues were the first to provide preclinical data supporting a potential role for VEGF gene transfer in the amelioration of ED. Most recently, others have shown the ability to utilize a nonviral gene transfer delivery system for VEGF in a diabetic rat model. Data from these studies demonstrate that VEGF gene therapy using this system could be useful in improving erectile function in diabetic men (60).

Because relaxation of corporal and arterial smooth muscle of the penis is key (in the absence of veno-occlusive dysfunction) to normal erectile capacity, many studies have also focused on gene transfer strategies to improve smooth muscle relaxation. In an excellent review, Burnett and colleagues summarize the strategies used (11), including the following: (a) antisense oligonucleotide strategies targeting PDE-5 and the NO/cGMP/PKG pathway (61); (b) modulation of other second messengers/receptors/effectors of arterial and corporal smooth muscle cell tone such as the cAMP pathway via calcitonin gene-related peptide (CGRP) and VIP, respectively (62, 63), the calcium sensitization pathway (i.e., RhoA/Rho-kinase pathway (64); and (c) ion channels, specifically the human large conductance, calcium-sensitive K channel (hSlo; the Maxi-K channel) (65) or the metabolically regulated K channel (i.e., KATP) (66) (Fig. 11.2).

Magee and colleagues were the first to investigate targeting of nNOS or the penile-specific variant of nNOS transfections in the rat model using a "gutless" (i.e., replication incompetent) adenovirus vector, as well as plasmids (68). The same group also evaluated the utility of pSilencer2.1-U6-PINshRNA gene therapy (protein inhibitor of nNOS [PIN]) and concluded that it was more effective than the antisense PIN mRNA in ameliorating ED in the aged rat (69).

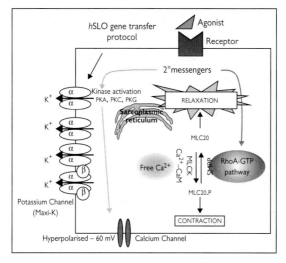

Figure 11.2 Insertion of Maxi-K channels into smooth muscle cell. A representative cell into which the a-subunit of the MaxiK channel has been transferred. Three additional MaxiK channels are shown in the cell membrane. MLC20, myosin light chain 20; MLCK, myosin light chain kinase; PKA, protein kinase A; PKC, protein kinase C; PKG, protein kinase G; SMPP, smooth muscle myosin phosphatase.[67]

Several studies have examined gene transfer with neurotrophic factors. Bakirciouglu and colleagues (70) examined the ability of brain-derived neurotrophic factor gene therapy to restore the cavernous nerve-stimulated intracavernous pressure response in a rat model of neurogenic impotence. Their results provide proof of concept that increasing the magnitude of the stimulus for erection can be accomplished via manipulation of neuronal innervation density. In another study, Kato and colleagues (71) used gene transfer with HSV expressing GDNF (or neurturin) in rats where the cavernous nerve was bilaterally injured using a clamp and dry ice. Four weeks after nerve injury, treated rats displayed significant recovery of erectile function compared with rats treated with control vector or untreated rats.

In 2003 the U.S. Food and Drug Administration approved the first trial of gene transfer to treat ED. The gene chosen was hSlo. The hSlo gene encodes the expression of the α, or pore-forming, unit of the large-conductance calcium (Ca) and voltage-activated potassium (K)-ion channel known as the BKCa, or Maxi-K, channel. The BKCa channel is composed of a tetramer of six membrane-spanning proteins that, when in the open state, selectively conduct K+ ions down the electrochemical gradient out of the cell at a rate of 106 to 108 ions/sec in all cells in the body except cardiomyocytes (72). This results in hyperpolarization of the cell and closure of voltage-dependent calcium channels that decrease Ca^{2+} entry into the cell. The inhibition of Ca^{2+} influx into vascular smooth muscle cells causes the smooth muscle cells to relax, with consequent vasodilatation. As a result, the K+ channels are required for maintenance of vascular tone as they counteract and balance vasoconstrictor events within the smooth muscle cells (73). The BKCa channels can considered as a natural feedback mechanism to oppose smooth muscle contractility. Alterations in K^+ channel physiology and function increasingly are being recognized as major contributing factors to the development of the vascular pathological conditions associated with diabetes and aging (74, 75). The first human clinical trial of gene transfer for the treatment of ED has been completed (76). In this seminal dose-escalation safety study, sponsored by Ion Channel Innovations, LLC (see http://www.ionchannelinnovations.com for details), 11 patients with moderate to severe ED were given a single corpus cavernosum injection of hMaxi-K, a "naked" DNA plasmid carrying the human cDNA encoding hSlo (for human slow-poke), the gene for the α, or pore-forming, subunit of the human smooth muscle Maxi-K channel (in a pVAX expression vector). No serious adverse events or dose-related adverse events attributed to gene transfer were observed for any patient at any dose during any study visit. In addition, secondary efficacy endpoints were measured using the International Index of Erectile Function (IIEF) scale, with patient responses validated by partner responses. In this regard these patients reported erectile function category improvements that were highly clinically significant and maintained throughout the 24 weeks of study. While efficacy conclusions clearly cannot be drawn from the results of a phase I trial, nonetheless these exciting data represent a major step toward one day making gene transfer a treatment option for ED.

Stem Cell and Cell-Based Therapies

Cellular therapy for the repair of damaged tissues and organs represents the entry-point technology for regenerative medicine. That is, in addition to technologies built around genetic modification of endogenous cells, another possibility is the (re)-implantation/introduction of cells into the corpus cavernosum, where the goal is to essentially "reseed" or "repopulate" the penis with the requisite cells for normal tissue/organ function. In theory, this could be accomplished by either systemic or intracorporal injection; however, direct injection is the currently preferred route of cellular delivery. Wessells and Williams (77) were the first to demonstrate the feasibility of utilizing autologous transplantation of endothelial cells into the corpus cavernosum of the rat for this purpose. Other researchers looked to utilize stem or progenitor cells. Stem cells, by definition, retain both their clonogenic capacity (i.e., ability for self-renewal) as well as their potential for multilineage differentiation (i.e., ability to differentiate into distinct cell types) (78). The use of autologous non–cell-line-induced adipose tissue-derived stem cells has shown promising early results for the treatment of ED. However, the mechanisms of action for stem cell therapy remain controversial, with increasing evidence supporting paracrine pathway mechanisms, and in the case of post-nerve injury ED, underlying mechanisms of recovery appear to involve neuron preservation and cytoprotection by inhibition of apoptosis (79). From a future therapy viewpoint, although there are limitations to the current fund of knowledge, this area of therapeutics holds particular promise (80).

Tissue Engineering for ED

At the other end of the regenerative medicine technology spectrum is tissue engineering. The basic concept is to use biocompatible, biodegradable scaffolds, either with or without cells, to repair damaged tissues and organs. The concept of tissue engineering in urology has received considerable attention recently and is especially attractive when the end-organ damage is very extensive, thus requiring replacement for restoration and maintenance of function (81–84). Regardless of the precise etiology for ED, it is clear that traditional pharmacotherapies will most likely eventually fail or will not provide satisfactory functional results (85). In these scenarios, the use of acellular scaffolds has shown value in preclinical studies for tunica patch repair (86) as well as cavernous nerve regeneration (87). Additionally, a number of studies have shown the usefulness of using tissue engineering for phallic reconstruction and formation and reconstitution of corporal tissue both in vitro and in vivo (88–92). In the example of phallic reconstruction, designed cartilage rods were combined with autologous chondrocytes suspended in biodegradable polymers. These structures were then implanted as processed penile prostheses and, remarkably, when retrieved had acquired biological characteristics of cartilage (88–91). These experiments demonstrate the likelihood of using autologous donor cells for corporal tissue reconstruction. Furthermore, human corporal smooth muscle and endothelial cells seeded on biodegradable scaffolds can form vascularized cavernosal tissue when implanted *in vivo* (90–92). In a rabbit model, this approach (autologous penile corpora cavernosa replacement) was sufficient to support mating activity by 3 months postoperatively (93). Development of methods to further enhance the cellular content, and thus function, of these engineered constructs are ongoing (94).

Conclusions

The rapid growth of basic science understanding underpins the development of future erectile restoration therapy. Given the wide scope of potential strategies, including novel pharmacotherapeutics, therapies involving growth factors, gene therapy, or stem cell and cell-based approaches, and regenerative medicine, we are confident that these areas of ongoing and future research will translate into safe, effective, and potentially curative therapies for ED.

References

1. Andersson KE, Wagner G. Physiology of penile erection. *Physiol Rev* 1995;75:191–236.

2. Burnett AL. Nitric oxide in the penis: Physiology and pathology. *J Urol* 1997;157:320–324.

3. Burnett AL. Nitric oxide in the penis—science and therapeutic implications from erectile dysfunction to priapism. *J Sex Med* 2006;3:578–582.

4. Toda N, Ayajiki K, Okamura T. Nitric oxide and penile erectile function. *Pharmacol Ther* 2005;106:233–266.

5. Hurt KJ, Sezen SF, Champion HC, Crone JK, Palese MA, Huang PL, Sawa A, Luo X, Musicki B, Snyder SH, Burnett AL. Alternatively spliced neuronal nitric oxide synthase mediates penile erection. *Proc Natl Acad Sci USA* 2006;103:3440–3443.

6. Hurt KJ, Musicki B, Palese MA, Crone JK, Becker RE, Moriarity JL, Snyder SH, Burnett AL. Akt-dependent phosphorylation of endothelial nitric-oxide synthase mediates penile erection. *Proc Natl Acad Sci USA* 2002;99:4061–4066.

7. Musicki B, Burnett AL. eNOS function and dysfunction in the penis. *Exp Biol Med (Maywood)* 2006;231:154–165.

8. Pfeifer A, Klatt P, Massberg S, Ny L, Sausbier M, Hirneiss C, Wang GX, Korth M, Aszódi A, Andersson KE, Krombach F, Mayerhofer A, Ruth P, Fässler R, Hofmann F. Defective smooth muscle regulation in cGMP kinase I-deficient mice. *EMBO J* 1998;17:3045–3051.

9. Sadeghipour H, Ghasemi M, Ebrahimi F, Dehpour AR. Effect of lithium on endothelium-dependent and neurogenic relaxation of rat corpus cavernosum: Role of nitric oxide pathway. *Nitric Oxide* 2007;16:54–63.

10. Hedlund P, Aszodi A, Pfeifer A, Alm P, Hofmann F, Ahmad M, Fassler R, Andersson KE. Erectile dysfunction in cyclic GMP-dependent kinase I-deficient mice. *Proc Natl Acad Sci USA* 2000;97:2349–2354.

11. Burnett AL et al. Future sexual medicine physiological treatment targets. *J Sex Med* 2010;7:3269–3304.

12. Bivalacqua TJ, Kendirci M, Champion HC, Hellstrom WJ, Andersson KE, Hedlund P. Dysregulation of cGMPdependent protein kinase 1 (PKG-1) impairs erectile function in diabetic rats: Influence of in vivo gene therapy of PKG1 alpha. *BJU Int* 2007;99:1488–1494.

13. Angulo J, Cuevas P, Fernández A, Allona A, Moncada I, Mart´n-Morales A, La Fuente JM, de Tejada IS. Enhanced thromboxane receptor-mediated responses and impaired endothelium-dependent relaxation in human corpus cavernosum from diabetic impotent men: Role of protein kinase C activity. *J Pharmacol Exp Ther* 2006;319:783–789.

14. Shamloul R. The potential role of the heme oxygenase/carbon monoxide system in male sexual dysfunctions. *J Sex Med* 2009;6:324–333.

15. Somlyo AP, Somlyo AV. Signal transduction by G-proteins, rho-kinase and protein phosphatase to smooth muscle and non-muscle myosin II. *J Physiol* 2000;15:177–185.

16. Fukata M, Kaibuchi K. Rho-family GTPases in cadherin mediated cell-cell adhesion. *Nat Rev Mol Cell Biol* 2001;2:887–897.

17. Jin L, Burnett Chitaley K, Webb RC, Mills TM. Rho-kinase as a potential target for the treatment of erectile dysfunction. *Drug News Perspect* 2001;14:601–606.

18. Jin L, Burnett AL. RhoA/Rho-kinase in erectile tissue: mechanisms of disease and therapeutic insights. *Clin Sci* 2006;110:153–165.

19. Vignozzi L, Morelli A, Filippi S, Ambrosini S, Mancina R, Luconi M, Mungai S, Vannelli GB, Zhang XH, Forti G, Maggi M. Testosterone regulates RhoA/Rho-kinase signalling in two distinct animal models of chemical diabetes. *J Sex Med* 2007;4:620–632.

20. Gao YT, Panda SP, Roman LJ, Martásek P, Ishimura Y, Masters BS. Oxygen metabolism by neuronal nitric-oxide synthase. *J Biol Chem* 2007;282:7921–7929.

21. Giuliano F, Allard J. Apomorphine SL (Uprima): preclinical and clinical experiences learned from the first central nervous system-acting ED drug. *Int J Impot Res* 2002;Suppl 1:S53–S56.

22. Hull EM, Warner RK, Bazzett TJ, Eaton RC, Thompson JT, Scaletta LL. D2/D1 ratio in the medial preoptic area affects copulation of male rats. *J Pharmacol Exp Ther* 1989;251:422–427.

23. Proctor JD, Chremos AN, Evans EF, Wasserman AJ. An apomorphine-induced vomiting model for antiemetic studies in man. *J Clin Pharmacol* 1978;18:95–99.

24. Andersson KE. Pharmacology of penile erection. *Pharmacol Rev* 2001;53:417–50.

25. Andersson KE. Neurophysiology/pharmacology of erection. *Int J Impot Res* 2001;13(3 suppl):S8–17.

26. Andersson KE. Pharmacology of erectile function and dysfunction. *Urol Clin North Am* 2001;28:233–247.

27. Andersson KE. Neurotransmitters: Central and peripheral mechanisms. Int J Impot Res 2000;12(4 suppl):S26–33.

28. Kim NN, Kim JJ, Hypolite J, Garc´a-D´az JF, Broderick GA, Tornheim K, Daley JT, Levin R, Saenz de Tejada I. Altered contractility of rabbit penile corpus caverno-sum smooth muscle by hypoxia. *J Urol* 1996;155:772–778.

29. Saenz de Tejada I, Carson MP, de las Morenas A, Goldstein I, Traish AM. Endothelin: Localization, synthesis, activity, and receptor types in human penile corpus cavernosum. *Am J Physiol* 1991;261:H1078–1085.

30. Kendirci M, Pradhan L, Trost L, Gur S, Chandra S, Agrawal KC, Hellstrom WJ. Peripheral mechanisms of erectile dysfunction in a rat model of chronic cocaine use. *Eur Urol* 2007;52:555–563.

31. Becker AJ, Uckert S, Stief CG, Truss MC, Hartmann U, Jonas U. Systemic and cavernosal plasma levels of endothelin (1–21) during different penile condi-tions in healthy males and patients with erectile dysfunction. *World J Urol* 2001;19:371–376.

32. El Melegy NT, Ali ME, Awad EM. Plasma levels of endothelin-1, angiotensin II, nitric oxide and prostaglandin E in the venous and cavernosal blood of patients with erectile dysfunction. *BJU Int* 2005;96:1079–1086.

33. Kim NN, Dhir V, Azadzoi KM, Traish AM, Flaherty E, Goldstein I. Pilot study of the endothelin-A receptor selective antagonist BMS-193884 for the treatment of erectile dysfunction. *J Androl* 2002;23:76–83.

34. Burnett AL. Erectile dysfunction management for the future. *J Androl* 2009;30:391–396.

35. Burnett AL, Lue TF. Neuromodulatory therapy to improve erectile function recovery outcomes after pelvic surgery. *J Urol* 2006;176:882–887.

36. Bella AJ, Lin G, Cagiannos I, Lue TF. Emerging neuromodulatory molecules for the treatment of neurogenic erectile dysfunction caused by cavernous nerve injury. *Asian J Androl* 2008;10:54–59.

37. Burgers JK, Nelson RJ, Quinlan DM, Walsh PC. Nerve growth factor, nerve grafts and amniotic membrane grafts restore erectile function in rats. *J Urol* 1991;146:463–468.

38. Ball RA, Lipton SA, Dreyer EB, Richie JP, Vickers MA. Entubulization repair of severed cavernous nerves in the rat resulting in return of erectile function. *J Urol* 1992;148:211–215.

39. Bella AJ, Lin G, Tantiwongse K, Garcia M, Lin CS, BrantW, Lue TF. Brain-derived neurotrophic factor (BDNF) acts primarily via the JAK/STAT pathway to pro-mote neurite growth in the major pelvic ganglion of the rat: Part I. *J Sex Med* 2006;3:815–820.

40. Lin G, Bella AJ, Lue TF, Lin CS. Brain-derived neurotrophic factor (BDNF) acts primarily via the JAK/STAT pathway to promote neurite growth in the major pelvic ganglion of the rat: Part 2. *J Sex Med* 2006;3:821–827.

41. Bella AJ, Lin G, Garcia MM, Tantiwongse K, Brant WO, Lin CS, Lue TF. Upregulation of penile brain-derived neurotrophic factor (BDNF) and activation

of the JAK/STAT signalling pathway in the major pelvic ganglion of the rat after cavernous nerve transection. *Eur Urol* 2007;52:574–580.

42. Steiner JP, Hamilton GS, Ross DT, Valentine HL, Guo H, Connolly MA, Liang S, Ramsey C, Li JH, Huang W, Howorth P, Soni R, Fuller M, Sauer H, Nowotnik AC, Suzdak PD. Neurotrophic immunophilin ligands stimulate structural and functional recovery in neurodegenerative animal models. *Proc Natl Acad Sci USA* 1997;94:2019–2024.

43. Gold BG. Neuroimmunophilin ligands: Evaluation of their therapeutic potential for the treatment of neurological disorders. *Exp Opin Invest Drugs* 2000;9:2331–2342.

44. Allaf ME, Hoke A, Burnett AL. Erythropoietin promotes the recovery of erectile function following cavernous nerve injury. *J Urol* 2005;174:2060–2064.

45. Burnett AL, Allaf ME, Bivalacqua TJ. Erythropoietin promotes erection recovery after nerve-sparing radical retropubic prostatectomy: A retrospective analysis. *J Sex Med* 2008;5:2392–2398.

46. Henry GD, Byrne R, Hunyh TT, Abraham V, Annex BH, Hagen PO, Donatucci CF. Intracavernosal injections of vascular endothelial growth factor protects endothelial dependent corpora cavernosal smooth muscle relaxation in the hypercholesterolemic rabbit: A preliminary study. *Int J Impot Res* 2000;12:334–339.

47. Burchardt M, Burchardt T, Anastasiadis AG, Buttyan R, de la Taille A, Shabsigh A, Frank J, Shabsigh R. Application of angiogenic factors for therapy of erectile dysfunction: Protein and DNA transfer of VEGF 165 into the rat penis. *Urology* 2005;66:665–670.

48. Byrne AM, Bouchier-Hayes DJ, Harmey JH. Angiogenic and cell survival functions of vascular endothelial growth factor (VEGF). *J Cell Mol Med* 2005;9:777–794.

49. Lin CS, Ho HC, Chen KC, Lin G, Nunes L, Lue TF. Intracavernosal injection of vascular endothelial growth factor induces nitric oxide synthase isoforms. *BJU Int* 2002;89:955–960.

50. Musicki B, Palese MA, Crone JK, Burnett AL. Phosphorylated endothelial nitric oxide synthase mediates vascular endothelial growth factor-induced penile erection. *Biol Reprod* 2004;70:282–289.

51. Carneiro FS, Zemse S, Giachini FR, Carneiro ZN, Lima VV, Webb RC, Tostes RC. TNF-alpha infusion impairs corpora cavernosa reactivity. *J Sex Med* 2009;6(3 suppl):311–319.

52. Saraswat P, Soni RR, Bhandari A, Nagori BP. DNA as therapeutics; an update. *Indian J Pharm Sci* 2009;71:488–498.

53. Ratko TA, Cummings JP, Blebea J, Matuszewski KA. Clinical gene therapy for nonmalignant disease. *Am J Med* 2003;115:560–569.

54. Melman A, Kelvin D. Gene therapy for erectile dysfunction: What is the future? *Davies Curr Urol Rep* 2010;11:421–426.

55. Koransky ML, Robbins RC, Blau HM. VEGF gene delivery for treatment of ischemic cardiovascular disease. *Trends Cardiovasc Med* 2002;12:108–114.

56. Lee MC, El-Sakka AI, Graziottin TM, Ho HC, Lin CS, Lue TF. The effect of vascular endothelial growth factor on a rat model of traumatic arteriogenic erectile dysfunction. *J Urol* 2002;167:761–767.

57. Gholami SS, Rogers R, Chang J, Ho HC, Grazziottin T, Lin CS, Lue TF. The effect of vascular endothelial growth factor and adeno-associated virus mediated brain derived neurotrophic factor on neurogenic and vasculogenic erectile dysfunction induced by hyperlipidemia. *J Urol* 2003;169:1577–1581.

58. Rogers RS, Graziottin TM, Lin CS, Kan YW, Lue TF. Intracavernosal vascular endothelial growth factor (VEGF) injection and adeno-associated virus-mediated

VEGF gene therapy prevent and reverse venogenic erectile dysfunction in rats. *Int J Impot Res* 2003;15:26–37.

59. Ryu JK, Cho CH, Shin HY, Song SU, Oh SM, Lee M, Piao S, Han JY, Kim IH, Koh GY, Suh JK. Combined angiopoietin-1 and vascular endothelial growth factor gene transfer restores cavernous angiogenesis and erectile function in a rat model of hypercholesterolemia. *Mol Ther* 2006;13:5–15.

60. Dall'era JE, Meacham RB, Mills JN, Koul S, Carlsen SN, Myers JB, Koul HK. Vascular endothelial growth factor (VEGF) gene therapy using a nonviral gene delivery system improves erectile function in a diabetic rat model. *Int J Impot Res* 2008;3:307–314.

61. Bai WJ, Hou SK, Wang XF, Yan Z, He PY, Deng QP, Hu XP, Guan KP. The effects of antisenes oligodeoxynucleotide on the cyclic nucleotide monophosphates in smooth muscle cells of human corpus cavernosum. *Zhonghua Nan Ke Xue* 2002;8:88–91.

62. Bivalacqua TJ, Champion HC, Abdel-Mageed AB, Kadowitz PJ, Hellstrom WJ. Gene transfer of prepro-calcitonin generelated peptide restores erectile function in the aged rat. *Biol Reprod* 2001;65:1371–1377.

63. Shen ZJ, Wang H, Lu YL, Zhou XL, Chen SW, Chen ZD. Gene transfer of vasoactive intestinal polypeptide into the penis improves erectile response in the diabetic rat. *BJU Int* 2005;95:890–894.

64. Chitaley K, Bivalacqua TJ, Champion HC, Usta MF, HellstromWJ, Mills TM, Webb RC. Adeno-associated viral gene transfer of dominant negative RhoA enhances erectile function in rats. *Biochem Biophys Res Commun* 2002;298:427–432.

65. Melman A, Biggs G, Davies K, ZhaoW, Tar MT, Christ GJ. Gene transfer with a vector expressing Maxi-K from a smooth muscle-specific promoter restores erectile function in the aging rat. *Gene Ther* 2008;15:364–370.

66. So I, Chae MR, Lee SW. Gene transfer of the K-ATP channel restores age-related erectile dysfunction in rats. *BJU Int J* 2007;100:1154–1160.

67. Melman A. Gene therapy for male erectile dysfunction. *Urol Clin North Am* 2007;34:619–630.

68. Magee TR, Ferrini M, Garban HJ, Vernet D, Mitani K, Rajfer J, Gonzalez-Cadavid NF. Gene therapy of erectile dysfunction in the rat with penile neuronal nitric oxide synthase. *Biol Reprod* 2002;67:1033–1041.

69. Magee TR, Kovanecz I, Davila HH, Ferrini MG, Cantini L, Vernet D, Zuniga FI, Rajfer J, Gonzalez-Cadavid NF. Antisense and short hairpin RNA (shRNA) constructs targeting PIN (protein inhibitor of NOS) ameliorate aging related erectile dysfunction in the rat. *J Sex Med* 2007;4:633–643.

70. Bakircioglu ME, Lin CS, Fan P, Sievert KD, Kan YW, Lue TF. The effect of adeno-associated virus mediated brain derived neurotrophic factor in an animal model of neurogenic impotence. *J Urol* 2001;165:2103–2109.

71. Kato R, Wolfe D, Coyle CH, Huang S, Wechuck JB, Goins WF, Krisky DM, Tsukamoto T, Nelson JB, Glorioso JC, Chancellor MB, Yoshimura N. Herpes simplex virus vectormediated delivery of glial cell line-derived neurotrophic factor rescues erectile dysfunction following cavernous nerve injury. *Gene Ther* 2007;14:1344–1352.

72. Shieh CC, Coghlan M, Sullivan JP, Gopalakrishnan M. Potassium channels: molecular defects, diseases, and therapeutic opportunities. *Pharmacol Rev* 2000;52:557–594.

73. Korovkina VP, England SK. Molecular diversity of vascular potassium channel isoforms. *Clin Exp Pharmacol Physiol* 2002;29:317–323.

74. Korovkina VP, England SK. Detection and implications of potassium channel alterations. *Vascul Pharmacol* 2002;38:3–12.

75. Davies KP, Zhao W, Tar M, et al.: Diabetes-induced changes in the alternative splicing of the slo gene in corporal tissue. *Eur Urol* 2007;52:1229–1237.

76. Melman A, Bar-Chama N, McCullough A, Davies K, Christ G. hMaxi-K gene transfer in males with erectile dysfunction: Results of the first human trial. *Hum Gene Ther* 2006;17:1165–76.

77. Wessells H, Williams SK. Endothelial cell transplantation into the corpus cavernosum: Moving towards cell-based gene therapy. *J Urol* 1999;162:2162–2164.

78. Rookmaaker MB, Verhaar MC, van Zonneveld AJ, Rabelink TJ. Progenitor cells in the kidney: Biology and therapeutic perspectives. *Kidney Int* 2004;66:518–522.

79. Albersen M, Fandel TM, Lin G, Wang G, Banie L, Lin CS, Lue TF. Injections of adipose tissue-derived stem cells and stem cell lysate improve recovery of erectile function in a rat model of cavernous nerve injury. *J Sex Med* 2010;7(10):3331–3340.

80. Strong TD, Gebska MA, Champion HC, Burnett AL, Bivalacqua TJ. Stem and endothelial progenitor cells in erection biology. *Int J Impot Res* 2008;20:243–254.

81. Wood D, Southgate J. Current status of tissue engineering in urology. *Curr Opin Urol* 2008;18:564–569.

82. Sievert KD, Amend B, Stenzl A. Tissue engineering for the lower urinary tract: A review of a state of the art approach. *Eur Urol* 2007;52:1580–1589.

83. Atala A, Bauer SB, Soker S, Yoo JJ, Retik AB. Tissue engineered autologous bladders for patients needing cystoplasty. *Lancet* 2006;367:1241–1246.

84. Atala A. Engineering tissues, organs and cells. *J Tissue Eng Regen Med* 2007;1:83–96.

85. Atala A. Engineering of cells and tissues for treatment of erectile dysfunction. *World J Urol* 2001;19:67–73.

86. Eberli D, Susaeta R, Yoo JJ, Atala A. Tunica repair with acellular bladder matrix maintains corporal tissue function. *Int J Impot Res* 2007;19:602–609.

87. Connolly SS, Yoo JJ, Abouheba M, Soker S, McDougal WS, Atala A. Cavernous nerve regeneration using acellular nerve grafts. *World J Urol* 2008;26:333–339.

88. Yoo JJ, Lee I, Atala A. Cartilage rods as a potential material for penile reconstruction. *J Urol* 1998;160:1164–1178.

89. Yoo JJ, Park HJ, Lee I, Atala A. Autologous engineered cartilage rods for penile reconstruction. *J Urol* 1999;162:1119–1121.

90. Yoo JJ, Park HJ, Atala A. Tissue-engineering applications for phallic reconstruction. *World J Urol* 2000;18:62–66.

91. Kershen RT, Yoo JJ, Moreland RB, Krane RJ, Atala A. Reconstitution of human corpus cavernosum smooth muscle in vitro and in vivo. *Tissue Eng* 2002;8:515–524.

92. Falke G, Yoo JJ, Kwon TG, Moreland R, Atala A. Formation of corporal tissue architecture in vivo using human cavernosal muscle and endothelial cells seeded on collagen matrices. *Tissue Eng* 2003;9:871–879.

93. Kwon TG, Yoo JJ, Atala A. Autologous penile corpora cavernosa replacement using tissue engineering techniques. *J Urol* 2002;168:1754–1758.

94. Eberli D, Susaeta R, Yoo JJ, Atala A. A method to improve cellular content for corporal tissue engineering. *Tissue Eng Part A* 2008;14:1581–1589.

Index